Integumentary Essentials

Applying the Preferred Physical Therapist Practice Patterns℠

Integumentary Essentials

Applying the Preferred Physical Therapist Practice Patterns^{SM}

Editor

Marilyn Moffat, PT, DPT, PhD, FAPTA, CSCS

Professor, Physical Therapy Department

New York University

New York, New York

Associate Editor

Katherine Biggs Harris, PT, MS

Assistant Professor in Physical Therapy

Quinnipiac University

Hamden, Connecticut

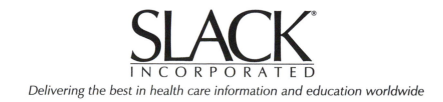

Delivering the best in health care information and education worldwide

BS

www.slackbooks.com

ISBN-10: 1-55642-670-4
ISBN-13: 978-1-55642-670-4

The procedures and practices described in this book should be implemented in a manner consistent with the professional standards set for the circumstances that apply in each specific situation. Every effort has been made to confirm the accuracy of the information presented and to correctly relate generally accepted practices. The authors, editor, and publisher cannot accept responsibility for errors or exclusions or for the outcome of the material presented herein. There is no expressed or implied warranty of this book or information imparted by it. Care has been taken to ensure that drug selection and dosages are in accordance with currently accepted/recommended practice. Due to continuing research, changes in government policy and regulations, and various effects of drug reactions and interactions, it is recommended that the reader carefully review all materials and literature provided for each drug, especially those that are new or not frequently used. Any review or mention of specific companies or products is not intended as an endorsement by the author or publisher.

SLACK Incorporated uses a review process to evaluate submitted material. Prior to publication, educators or clinicians provide important feedback on the content that we publish. We welcome feedback on this work.

Some material contained in this book is reprinted with permission from the American Physical Therapy Association. *Guide to Physical Therapist Practice.* 2nd ed. Alexandria, Va: APTA; 2001 and appears courtesy of the APTA. For more information, please contact the APTA directly at www.apta.org.

Published by: SLACK Incorporated
                 6900 Grove Road
                 Thorofare, NJ 08086 USA
                 Telephone: 856-848-1000
                 Fax: 856-853-5991
                 www.slackbooks.com

Contact SLACK Incorporated for more information about other books in this field or about the availability of our books from distributors outside the United States.

Library of Congress Cataloging-in-Publication Data

Integumentary essentials: applying the preferred physical therapist practice patterns / editor, Marilyn Moffat; associate editor, Katherine Biggs Harris.

  p. ; cm. -- (Essentials in physical therapy)
Includes bibliographical references and index.
ISBN-13: 978-1-55642-670-4 (alk. paper)
ISBN-10: 1-55642-670-4 (alk. paper)
1. Skin--Diseases--Physical therapy. 2. Skin--Diseases--Patients--Rehabilitation. I. Moffat, Marilyn. II. Harris, Katherine Biggs. II. Series.
  [DNLM: 1. Skin Diseases--therapy--Case Reports. 2. Patient Care Planning--Case Reports. 3. Physical Therapy Modalities--standards--Case Reports. WR 140 I595 2006]
  RL110.I52 2006
  616.5--dc22

Printed in the United States of America.

Last digit is print number: 10 9 8 7 6 5 4 3 2 1

5/1/07

Dedication

Undertaking a task of this magnitude is never possible without the utmost support of many individuals to whom I am deeply indebted. Thus this book is dedicated to: all of my Moffat and Salant families; physical therapy colleagues; APTA staff; faculty, support staff, and students at New York University; and all of my patients and clients who made this endeavor possible.

—MM

To my many colleagues, students, patients, and their families...
you have provided me with so many learning and teaching opportunities.
To my family, Buck, Stephanie, Mom (Grace), and Dad (Peter)...
for your constant support in all my endeavors.

—KBH

Contents

Acknowledgments

This edited book is one of a series of four books that would not have been possible without the dedication, incredibly hard work, and generosity of so many individuals. I am eternally indebted to each of the following outstanding physical therapists for their willingness to share their expertise, their enthusiasm, and their unbelievable patience in seeing this work come to fruition:

- ♦ Associate Editor:
  - Katherine Biggs Harris, PT, MS
- ♦ Contributing Authors:
  - Katherine Biggs Harris, PT, MS
  - Jenna Driscoll, PT, MS
  - Betsy A. Myers, PT, MPT, MHS, OCS, CLT
  - Carrie Sussman, PT, DPT

The putting together of a book requires the astute skills of both editorial and publishing staff. Working with colleagues and associates at SLACK Incorporated has indeed been a pleasure, and I am indebted to them for their perceptive reviews and their continued encouragement provided along the way. To the following individuals I owe my thanks:

- ♦ Carrie Kotlar, who first approached me with the idea of doing this book and stood by throughout the process with unwavering support
- ♦ John Bond, who jumped in whenever we needed support from the top
- ♦ Jennifer Cahill and Kimberly Shigo, who had the editorial tasks of making our manuscripts into a published book

And last, but not least, are so many who have influenced my life, have challenged me to strive to do the best that I am able, and have supported and encouraged me along the way. My heartfelt thanks are extended to:

- ♦ My mother, for her unconditional support
- ♦ My father and my husband who were always there for me, were both the epitome of role models, and were both taken from me too early in life
- ♦ My sister and brother-in-law, my stepdaughter, and my grandchildren for always reminding me of what is important in life
- ♦ All of my physical therapy colleagues, who have been such an integral part of my life
- ♦ The staff at the American Physical Therapy Association, who continually supported me throughout the years and who sometimes met unbelievable demands to see the *Guide* project reach the format it is today
- ♦ The faculty and support staff at New York University, my students, and my patients who have taught me so much and made me realize what insight and passion mean in realizing one's goals

Setting an example is not the main means of influencing others; it is the only means—Albert Einstein

—*MM*

I would like to thank Marilyn Moffat for the opportunity to write and edit this book. My colleagues, Betsy, Carrie, and Jenna, for making this book a reality…thank you. Without your assistance, guidance, and support this would not have been possible. And finally, many thanks to Carrie and Jennifer at SLACK Incorporated for their constant availability and assistance during this process…you have been wonderful.

—*KBH*

About the Editors

Marilyn Moffat, PT, DPT, PhD, FAPTA, CSCS, a recognized leader in the United States and internationally, is a practitioner, a teacher, a consultant, a leader, and an author. She received her baccalaureate degree from Queens College and her physical therapy certificate and PhD degrees from New York University. She is a Full Professor of Physical Therapy at New York University, where she directs both the professional doctoral program (DPT) and the post-professional graduate master's degree program in pathokinesiology. She has been in private practice for more than 40 years and currently practices in the New York area.

Dr. Moffat was one of the first individuals to speak and write about the need for a doctoral entry-level degree in physical therapy. Her first presentation on this topic was given to the Section for Education in 1977.

Dr. Moffat completed a 6-year term as the President of the American Physical Therapy Association (APTA) in 1997. Prior to that she had served on the APTA Board of Directors for 6 years and also as President of the New York Physical Therapy Association for 4 years. During her term as President of the APTA, she played a major role in the development of the Association's *Guide to Physical Therapist Practice* and was project editor of the Second Edition of the *Guide*. Among her many publications is the *American Physical Therapy Association's Book of Body Maintenance and Repair*. As part of her commitment to research, Dr. Moffat serves as a member of the Board of Trustees of the Foundation for Physical Therapy, was a previous member of the Financial Advisory Committee, and has done major fundraising for them over the years.

She is currently on the Executive Committee of the World Confederation for Physical Therapy (WCPT) as the North American/Caribbean Regional Representative, and she was a member of the WCPT Task Force to develop an international definition of physical therapy. She coordinated the efforts to develop international standards for physical therapist education and for physical therapy practice around the world. She has given more than 800 professional presentations throughout her practice lifetime, and she has taught and provided consultation services in Taiwan, Thailand, Burma, Vietnam, Panama City, Hong Kong, and Puerto Rico.

Her diversified background is exemplified by the vast number of APTA and New York Physical Therapy Association committees and task forces on which she has served or chaired. She has served as Editor of *Physical Therapy*, the official publication of the Association. She was also instrumental in the early development of the TriAlliance of Rehabilitation Professionals, composed of the APTA, the American Occupational Therapy Association, and the American Speech-Language-Hearing Association. She has been an Associate of the Council of Public Representatives of the National Institutes of Health.

Dr. Moffat is a Catherine Worthingham Fellow of the APTA. She has been the recipient of APTA's Marilyn Moffat Leadership Award; the WCPT's Mildred Elson Award for International Leadership; the APTA's Lucy Blair Service Award; the Robert G. Dicus Private Practice Section APTA Award for contributions to private practice; Outstanding Service Awards from the New York Physical Therapy Association and from the APTA; the Ambassador Award from the National Strength and Conditioning Association; the Howard A. Rusk Humanitarian Award from the World Rehabilitation Fund; the United Cerebral Palsy Citation for Service; the Sawadi Skulkai Lecture Award from Mahidol University in Bangkok, Thailand; New York University's Founders Day Award; the University of Florida's Barbara C. White Lecture Award; the Massachusetts General's Ionta Lecture Award; the Chartered Society of Physiotherapist's Alan Walker Memorial Lecture Award; the APTA Minority Affairs Diversity 2000 Award; and the Section of Health Policy's R. Charles Harker Policy Maker Award. In addition, the New York Physical Therapy Association also named its leadership award after her. She was the APTA's 2004 Mary McMillan Lecturer, the Association's highest award. Dr. Moffat has been listed in *Who's Who in the East, Who's Who in American Women, Who's Who in America, Who's Who in Education, Who's Who in the World*, and *Who's Who in Medicine and Healthcare*.

She is also currently on the Board of Directors of the World Rehabilitation Fund and is a member of the Executive Committee. In addition to her professional associations, she was elected to be a member of Kappa Delta Pi and Pi Lambda Theta.

Dr. Moffat has served on a Citizen's Advisory Council of the New York State Assembly Task Force on the Disabled, has been a member of the State Board for Physical Therapy in New York, has served as a consultant to the New York City Police Department, and has been a member of the Boards of Trustees of Children's Village and the Four Oaks Foundation. The Nassau County Fine Arts Museum, the Howard A. Rusk Rehabilitation Medicine Campaign Committee, Saint John's Church of Lattingtown, and the Nassau County American Red Cross have been the recipients of her volunteer services.

Katherine Biggs Harris, PT, MS, has been working in the area of integumentary disruption for more than 20 years. During this time she has been involved in patient care, teaching, and research. She received her baccalaureate degree from Russell Sage College; her master's degree in Research, Measurement, and Quantitative Analysis for the Behavioral Sciences and Education from Southern Connecticut State University; and is currently enrolled in a PhD program at Nova Southeastern University. She anticipates completion of her dissertation in 2007. Mrs. Harris is an Assistant Professor of Physical Therapy at Quinnipiac University. She continues to practice clinically at Yale New Haven Hospital as a per diem therapist.

Mrs. Harris has been professionally active at the state and national levels. She was President of the Connecticut Physical Therapy Association, Chairperson of the Committee on Chapters and Sections for the APTA, Chairperson of the Advisory Panel on Practice of the APTA, and a task force member for the *Guide to Physical Therapist Practice* Integumentary Preferred Practice Patterns and Tests and Measures.

Mrs. Harris has published in the *Journal of Burn Care and Rehabilitation, Acute Care Perspectives,* and the *Connecticut Physical Therapy Association Newsletter.* She has presented at numerous national, regional, and local meetings on integumentary management, critical care management, and use of evidence in practice.

Contributing Authors

Katherine Biggs Harris, PT, MS
Assistant Professor in Physical Therapy
Quinnipiac University
Hamden, Connecticut

Jenna Driscoll, PT, MS
Level III Therapist
Yale New Haven Hospital
New Haven, Connecticut

Betsy A. Myers, PT, MPT, MHS, OCS, CLT
Physical Therapist
St. John Health System
Tulsa, Oklahoma

Carrie Sussman, PT, DPT
Sussman Physical Therapy, Inc.
Torrance, California

Preface

Integumentary Essentials: Applying the Preferred Physical Therapist Practice Patterns^{SM} is part of a series of four books (*Musculoskeletal Essentials, Neuromuscular Essentials, Cardiovascular Essentials,* and *Integumentary Essentials*) aimed at promoting an understanding of physical therapist practice and challenging the clinical thinking and decision making of our practitioners. In this book, four distinguished contributors have written chapters to take the *Guide to Physical Therapist Practice* to the next level of practice. Each chapter provides the relevant information for the pattern described by the *Guide* and emphasizes the process through which a physical therapist goes to take the patient from the examination to discharge. The Introduction to this book describes what each chapter contains.

It has been a goal of this entire series, and certainly is a strong hope of each of us involved in editing this series, that these *Essentials* will provide students and practitioners with a valuable reference for physical therapist practice.

As a way of introduction to the *Guide to Physical Therapist Practice*, the information below provides a brief overview of its development. Since I was involved in each step of the entire process, I know the unbelievable amount of work done by so many to see that landmark work reach fruition.

DEVELOPMENT OF THE *GUIDE*

The *Guide to Physical Therapist Practice* was developed based on the needs of membership by the American Physical Therapy Association (APTA) under my leadership as President of the Association. As an integral part of all of the groups responsible for writing the *Guide* and as one of three Project Editors for the latest edition of the *Guide*, I was delighted when SLACK Incorporated approached me to take the *Guide* to the next step for students and clinicians.

HISTORY

In the way of history, the development of the *Guide* began in 1992 with a Board of Directors-appointed task force upon which I served and culminated in the publication of *A Guide to Physical Therapist Practice, Volume I: A Description of Patient Management* in the August 1995 issue of *Physical Therapy*. The APTA House of Delegates approved the development of Volume II, which was designed to describe the preferred patterns of practice for patient/client groupings commonly referred for physical therapy.

In 1997, Volume I and Volume II became Part One and Part Two of the *Guide*, and the first edition of the *Guide* was published in the November 1997 issue of *Physical Therapy*. In 1998, APTA began the development of Parts Three and Four of the *Guide* to catalog the specific tests and measures used by physical therapists in the four system areas and the areas of outcomes, health-related quality of life, and patient/client satisfaction. Additional inclusions in the *Guide* were standardized documentation forms and templates that incorporated the patient/client management process and a patient/client satisfaction instrument.

A CD-ROM version of the *Guide* was developed that included not only Part One and Part Two, but also the varied tests and measures used in practice along with their reliability and validity.

FIVE ELEMENTS OF PATIENT/CLIENT MANAGEMENT

The patient/client management model includes the five essential elements of examination, evaluation, diagnosis, prognosis, and intervention that result in optimal outcomes. The patient/client management process is dynamic and allows the physical therapist to progress the patient/client in the process, return to an earlier element for further analysis, or exit the patient/client from the process when the needs of the patient/client cannot be addressed by the physical therapist. The patient/client management process incorporates the disablement model (pathology/pathophysiology, impairments, functional limitations) throughout the five elements and outcomes, but also includes all aspects of risk reduction/prevention; health, wellness, and fitness; societal resources; and patient/client satisfaction. This is the physical therapist's clinical decision-making model.

APPLICATION OF THE *GUIDE* TO CLINICAL PRACTICE

The *Guide* has its practice patterns grouped according to each of the four systems—musculoskeletal, neuromuscular, cardiovascular/pulmonary, and integumentary. Thus, this *Essentials in Physical Therapy* series continues where the *Guide* leaves off and brings the *Guide* to meaningful, clinically based examples of each of the patterns. In each chapter in each system area, an overview of the pertinent anatomy, physiology, pathophysiology, imaging, and pharmacology is presented; then three case studies are presented for each pattern. Each case initially details the physical therapist examination, including the history, systems review, and tests and measures selected for that case. Then the evaluation, diagnosis, and prognosis and plan of care for the case are presented. Prior to the specific interventions for the case is the rationale for the interventions based on the available literature, thus ensuring that, when possible, the interventions are evidence-based. The anticipated goals and expected outcomes for the interventions are put forth as much as possible in functional and measurable terms. Finally, any special considerations for reexamination, discharge, and psychological aspects are delineated.

Foreword
to the *Essentials in*
Physical Therapy Series

There are many leaders, many educators, and some visionaries, but only a very special few individuals have all three characteristics. The Editor of this series of books, Dr. Marilyn Moffat, certainly has demonstrated these traits and is again helping to guide the profession of physical therapy, as well as all therapists, to a new level of cognitive analysis when implementing and effectively using the *Guide to Physical Therapist Practice*.

Dr. Moffat's dream was for the American Physical Therapy Association to develop the original *Guide*. She nurtured its birth, as well as its development. In 2001, the second edition and evolution of additional practice patterns was introduced to the profession. Although the *Guide* lays the foundation for the entire diagnostic process used by a physical therapist as a movement specialist, many colleagues have difficulty bridging the gap between this model for the entire patient management process and its application to an individual consumer of physical therapy services. Through Dr. Moffat's vision, she recognized this gap and has again tried to link the highest standard of professional process to the patient/client and his or her specific needs.

When you take the leadership of the Editor and combine that with the expertise and clinical mastery of the various chapter authors, the quality of these texts already sets the highest standard of literary reference for an experienced, novel, or student physical therapist.

There are few individuals who could or would take on this dedicated process that will widen the therapist's comprehension of a very difficult and complex process. Dr. Moffat has again contributed, in her typical scholarly fashion, to the world of physical therapy literature and to each practitioner's role as a service provider of health care around the world.

—*Darcy Umphred, PT, PhD, FAPTA*
University of the Pacific
Stockton, California

Foreword
to *Integumentary Essentials*

There are many leaders, many educators, and some visionaries within the practice of physical therapy. Dr. Marilyn Moffat has certainly demonstrated these traits. Her colleague Katherine Biggs Harris, a member of the original integumentary panel, who coordinated *Integumentary Essentials*, also exemplifies these traits.

As it is so aptly stated in the American Physical Therapy Association's *Guide to Physical Therapist Practice*, "The physical therapist practice addresses the needs of both patients and clients through a continuum of service across all delivery settings by identifying health improvement opportunities, providing interventions for existing and emerging problems, preventing or reducing the risk of additional complications, and promoting wellness and fitness to enhance human performance as it relates to movement and health." Having had the pleasure of serving on the original integumentary panel for writing the *Guide*, I have a true appreciation of its intended use. However, many of our therapist colleagues have difficulty bridging the gap between the entire patient management model and its application to an individual consumer of physical therapy services.

The integumentary system has many factors that contribute to the physical therapist's diagnostic process, particularly the disease/pathological process, the interpretation of diagnostic data, and the associated functional limitations. The *Guide* provides a comprehensive template for the primary provider of health care with the expectation of empowering the patient to regain functional movement and activities that are important to the patient, family, and/or caregivers. Specific to the integumentary system is need for prevention and risk factor reduction.

As you review the *Integumentary Essentials* chapters, there are four patterns that are identified by the depth of tissue loss. The fifth pattern addresses the specific issues related to risk and prevention. Each chapter addresses the evaluation tools and their interpretation, as well as specific clinical examples. These examples demonstrate the direct correlation to an interruption of the integumentary system and loss of function. The examples also demonstrate the need to interact and practice in collaboration with a variety of professionals.

The authors who have assisted Dr. Moffat in this book are experts in integumentary issues and provide examples demonstrating their clinical mastery.

This text is a phenomenal reference for the experienced or student physical therapist. It is a wonderful addition to physical therapy literature, providing an excellent example of the physical therapist's role in the management of integumentary issues.

—Pamela G. Unger, PT, CWS
The Center for Advanced Wound Care
Reading, Pennsylvania

Introduction

The chapters in *Integumentary Essentials* take the *Guide to Physical Therapist Practice*[1] to the next level and parallel the patterns in the *Guide*.

INTRODUCTORY INFORMATION

In each case, where appropriate, a review of the pertinent anatomy, physiology, pathophysiology, imaging, and pharmacology is provided as a means of background material.

PHYSICAL THERAPIST EXAMINATION

Each pattern details three case studies appropriate to that pattern in *Guide* format. Thus, the case begins with the physical therapist examination, which is divided into the three parts of the examination—the history, the systems review, and the specific tests and measures selected for that particular case.

HISTORY

The history provides the first information that will be obtained from the patient/client. The history is a crucial first step in the clinical decision-making process as it enables the physical therapist to form an early hypothesis that helps guide the remainder of the clinical examination. The interview with the patient/client and a review of other available information provide the initial facts upon which further testing will be done to determine the concerns, goals, and eventual plan of care.

SYSTEMS REVIEW

After the history has been completed, the next aspect of the examination is the systems review, which is comprised of a quick screen of the four systems areas and a screen of the communication, affect, cognition, language, and learning style. The cardiovascular/pulmonary review includes assessment of blood pressure, edema, heart rate, and respiratory rate. The integumentary review includes assessing for the presence of any scar formation, the skin color, and the skin integrity. The musculoskeletal review includes assessment of gross range of motion, gross strength, gross symmetry, height, and weight. The neuromuscular review consists of an assessment of gross coordinated movements (eg, balance, locomotion, transfers, and transitions). The screen for communication, affect, cognition, language, and learning style includes an assessment of the patient's/client's ability to make needs known, consciousness, expected emotional/behavioral responses, learning preferences, and orientation.

TESTS AND MEASURES

The specific tests and measures to be selected for the patient/client are based upon the results found during the history taking and during the systems review. These latter two portions of the examination identify the clinical indicators for pathology/pathophysiology, impairments, functional limitations, disabilities, risk factors, prevention, and health, wellness, and fitness needs that will enable one to select the most appropriate tests and measures for the patient/client.

EVALUATION, DIAGNOSIS, AND PROGNOSIS AND PLAN OF CARE

The next step in the patient/client management model is evaluation. All of the data obtained from the examination (history, systems review, and tests and measures) are analyzed and synthesized to determine the diagnosis, prognosis, and plan of care for the patient/client. Then, once the evaluation has been completed and all data have been analyzed, the diagnosis for the patient/client and the pattern(s) into which the patient/client fits are determined.

After a review of the prognosis statement, of the expected range of number of visits per episode, and of the factors that may modify the frequency of visits for the pattern in the *Guide*, the prognosis is determined. Mutually established outcomes and the interventions for the patient/client are determined.

In each case the *Guide* has set the expected course of visits for the patient/client (see Expected Range of Number of Visits Per Episode of Care in each pattern in the *Guide*). This range should be appropriate for 80% of the population. Any additional impairment(s) found during the examination may or may not increase the number of expected visits. There are many factors that may modify the frequency or duration of visits. These may include: the patient's/client's adherence to the program set by the physical therapist, the type and amount of social support and caregiver expertise, the patient's/client's level of impairment, the patient's/client's health insurance plan, and the patient's/client's overall health status. Each patient/client must be looked at individually when determining the frequency and duration of visits.

INTERVENTIONS

Through all the information gathered in the examination and evaluation and with the diagnosis, prognosis, and plan of care in place, the specific interventions for this patient/client are selected. Whenever possible, interventions that have been shown to be effective through high-quality scientific research are utilized. At the end of all of the interventions is a composite section on anticipated goals and expected outcomes.

REEXAMINATION AND DISCHARGE

Reexamination will be performed throughout the episode of care, particularly as the setting of care changes. Discharge will occur when anticipated goals and expected outcomes have been attained.

PSYCHOLOGICAL ASPECTS

For each case, psychological aspects are important to consider when attempting to motivate patients/clients to comply with a long-range intervention program of exercise and functional training. Among these considerations for all patterns are:

- ◆ Behavior is governed by expectancies and incentives
- ◆ The likelihood that people adopt a health behavior depends on three perceptions:
  - The perception that health is threatened
  - The expectancy that their behavioral change will reduce the threat
  - The expectancy that they are competent to change the behavior

It is necessary for physical therapists to understand reasons for noncompliance and formulate intervention plans accordingly. The number one indicator of future noncompliance is past poor compliance. Any psychological considerations beyond these in a particular case will be further detailed in that case.

PATIENT/CLIENT SATISFACTION

And finally for each case, the patient/client satisfaction with the physical therapy management would be determined by using the standard Patient/Client Satisfaction Questionnaire found in the back of the *Guide*.

REFERENCES

1. American Physical Therapy Association. Guide to physical therapist practice. 2nd ed. *Phys Ther*. 2001;81:9-744.

CHAPTER ONE

Primary Prevention/ Risk Reduction for Integumentary Disorders (Pattern A)

Katherine Biggs Harris, PT, MS

ANATOMY

The skin is one of the largest functioning organs of the body.[1-3] The skin offers protection from the environment, in particular bacteria. The skin prevents the loss of body fluids, synthesizes vitamin D, and assists in temperature regulation. Other functions of the integument include its function as an excretory organ and a sensory organ.[4] Finally, the skin offers a component of one's identity.[3]

The skin is a layered system compromised of the epidermis, the dermis, and the subcutaneous layers (Figure 1-1). The epidermis, the thinner outermost layer of the skin, is made of the following layers. The stratum corneum, also known as the horny layer, is the outermost layer of the skin. This layer is composed of keratinocytes that have completely elongated and lost their nuclei. This layer is important for protection and acts as a barrier to external threats, such as bacteria. Keratinocytes reproduce continually and are responsible for the production of keratin, a protein that is insoluble in water. These cells prevent loss of water and offer protection from irritants and microorganisms.[2,4] The next layer is known as the stratum lucidum. This layer contains a few layers of flattened, dead keratinocytes.[2] The stratum granulosum or granular layer is found beneath the stratum lucidum. This layer is also composed of layers of flattened keratinocytes and significant amounts of keratin.[3] The next

layer is the stratum spinosum or spinous layer. This layer contains mature keratinocytes that appear "spiny" when observed under a microscope.[3,4] The final layer found is the stratum basale or basal cell layer. This layer is a cell layer of keratinocytes that are continually dividing and migrating upward to form the outer functional layers of the epidermis.[3,4] The stratum basale is attached to the dermis by the basement membrane.[3] Additional microscopic components of the epidermis include melanocytes and Langerhans' cells.[1-4] Melanocytes are found near the base of the epidermis. These cells synthesize and secrete melanin.[1-4] Melanin is the pigment one sees when observing the skin. Langerhans' cells are immune cells, are present throughout the epidermis, and initiate an immune response if the integument is disrupted, thus acting as a defense mechanism against the environment.[4]

The second layer of the skin is the thicker layer in comparison to the epidermis and is referred to as the dermis or dermal layer.[4] The dermis is further differentiated into the papillary dermis and the reticular dermis. The papillary dermis consists of a gel-like substance, also known as ground substance. The papillary dermis assists the basement membrane in creating the epidermal-dermal junction. The deeper reticular dermis is a connective tissue composed of fibroblasts that secrete collagen and elastin.[3] This gives the skin its elasticity and durability. This layer contains a significant

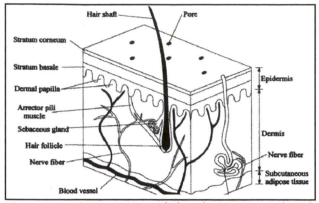

Figure 1-1. Components of the skin. Reprinted with permission from Irion G. *Comprehensive Wound Management*. Thorofare, NJ: SLACK Incorporated; 2002:4.

number of structures that include capillaries, lymph vessels, and nerve endings.[1] The dermis also contains hair follicles, sebaceous glands, and sweat glands that are often referred to as dermal appendages.[1] These structures are important in the regeneration of new epidermis following injury.[5]

The subcutaneous tissue, also known as the hypodermis, lies beneath the epidermis and dermis and supports these structures. It consists of fat or adipose tissue, connective tissue, and elastic tissue. The subcutaneous layer offers cushioning and insulation for the rest of the body.[1,4]

MICROSCOPIC STRUCTURES

Skin consists of a number of microscopic structures that include melanocytes, which are the dendritic cells that produce the pigment melanin and are found in the epidermal layer. Another type of cell found in the epidermal layer is the Langerhans' cell. These are also a type of dendritic cell and assist in the initial immune response if the skin has been disrupted.[4,5] Langerhans' cells are also responsible for the ultimate rejection of allograft skin when used as a temporary coverage. Finally, Merkel cells are also found in the epidermis and may function as mechanoreceptors.[4,5]

Mast cells and macrophages reside in the dermal layer of the skin. Mast cells are responsible for the release of histamine necessary during the inflammatory response phase of wound healing. Macrophages are also located throughout the dermis and are responsible for the phagocytosis of dead cells and other microorganisms that may penetrate the skin.[2]

The dermal appendages, hair follicles, sebaceous glands, and sweat glands are lined with epithelium but reside in the dermal layer and assist in epidermal resurfacing after partial-thickness injuries of the integument.[5] Finally, there is a layer of smooth muscle known as the arrector pilorum that inserts onto the connective tissue sheath of a hair follicle, causing "goosebumps."[6]

PHYSIOLOGY

The skin undergoes keratinocyte production and the desquamation of the outer layers of the stratum corneum that is normal epidermal regeneration.[5] Injury to the integument initiates a series of overlapping phases—the inflammatory phase, the proliferative phase, and the maturation phase—to promote wound healing.[3,5] Acute injury to the skin initiates an inflammatory response that typically lasts from 3 to 7 days and includes the following processes that are a combination of vascular and cellular responses. First, there is a vascular response to the injury that includes initial vasoconstriction to slow blood loss in the area. This immediate response only lasts a few minutes and is mediated by norepinephrine. During this phase of immediate vasoconstriction, a parallel process is also occurring, that of neutrophilic margination. Neutrophilic margination is seen as leukocytes begin to adhere to the injured endothelium.[3,5]

Vasodilatation occurs next and is noted for an increase in endothelial wall permeability to allow plasma proteins and leukocyte migration to occur. The cellular response involved is that of neutrophils being attracted to the area of injury and beginning the process of phagocytosis.[5] Phagocytosis is the process by which bacteria and debris are engulfed and destroyed.[3] Monocytes arrive next and once they are in interstitium they are known as macrophages.[5] Macrophages assist in the regulation of the inflammatory response as well as in decontamination.[3,5]

Finally, chemical mediators are involved in the inflammatory process. Their role ranges from protagonists to antagonists, and some may be synergistic. These chemical mediators include histamine, serotonin, kinins, prostaglandins, a number of proteins called the complement system, and growth factors. These chemical mediators continue to be investigated to determine their precise role in wound healing, specifically the inflammatory phase.[5]

Clinical manifestations of the inflammatory phase include swelling, redness, heat, and pain. The combination of pain and swelling can also create a reduction or loss of function.[7]

The second phase of wound healing is known as the proliferative phase or collagen phase.[8] This phase continues until the wound has resurfaced or healed.[3] Healing may occur via two pathways: regeneration or repair. Regeneration is seen when wound healing occurs via epithelialization or new skin formation. Repair is wound healing that involves granulation tissue formation, wound contraction, and epithelialization.[3,5] Repair may also occur through surgical interventions and these will be discussed in Pattern E: Impaired Integumentary Integrity Associated With Skin Involvement Extending Into Fascia, Muscle, or Bone and Scar Formation.

Re-epithelialization or resurfacing of the epidermis may occur in several ways. Epidermal cells have the potential to migrate from the wound edges in a "train" fashion allowing for resurfacing. Dermal appendages, which are lined with epithelial cells, may also assist with re-epithelialization as the cells migrate to the surface of the defect and create "islands" of epithelium.[3,5]

Wounds that extend into the dermis may heal by regeneration or repair depending on the degree of tissue destruction. Wounds that extend into the deeper dermis produce granulation tissue. Granulation tissue consists of new blood vessels, fibroblasts, and ground substance. Ground substance is a gel-like substance secreted by the fibroblasts. Granulation tissue is eventually replaced by scar.[5]

As wounds continue to granulate, wound contracture also begins to occur as a result of myofibroblasts that are transformed into fibroblasts that attempt to pull the wound together. Wound closure occurs as a result of granulation, contraction, and eventual epithelialization from the wound periphery.

The third and final phase of wound healing is considered the maturation phase or remolding phase. This phase of collagen reorganization occurs as early as 2 weeks post-injury. Collagen reorganization includes shrinking and thinning of the collagen laid down.[3-5] Contraction occurs to allow for wound closure, and as maturation progresses, the risk for contracture exists. Contracture is the possible result of contraction and should be monitored throughout the healing process.[7] There are also abnormal results of collagen reorganization. They include keloid scar formation and hypertrophic scar formation. Keloid scar formation is characterized by scar formation that extends beyond the borders of the original injury. Hypertrophic scarring is also considered abnormal scarring, but the excessive scar formation remains within the boundaries of the original injury.[4] Hypertrophic scarring has the potential to be modified through chemical and mechanical means[3] that will be discussed within the various case studies in subsequent chapters.

Acute injuries go through the overlapping phases of wound healing including inflammation, proliferation, and maturation. Wounds that exist in the proliferative phase for a period that extends beyond the normal time frames heal through a process considered chronic wound healing.[9]

Many wounds healing by secondary intention may become indolent. Lazarus defines chronic wounds as those that have "failed to proceed through an orderly and timely process to produce anatomic and functional integrity, or proceeded through the repair process without establishing a sustained anatomic and functional result."[10] Orderly refers to the orderly progression of the wound through the biological sequences that comprise the phases of repair. Orderliness may be interrupted during any of the phases of healing, but only recently are the causative factors for these interruptions being identified. Timeliness relates to the progression of the phases of repair proceeding in a manner that will heal the wound expeditiously. Timeliness is determined by the nature of the wound pathology, the medical status of the patient with the wound, and environmental factors. Those wounds that do not repair themselves in an orderly and timely manner are classified as chronic wounds. Chronic wounds have been recognized to have their own separate clinico-pathophysiologic entity.[11] Understanding of the clinico-pathophysiology of chronic wounds is a work in progress. A new model for chronic wound healing is developing. Chronic or nonhealing wounds are characterized as having prolonged inflammation, defective remodeling of the extracellular matrix (ECM), and failure to re-epithelialize.[9]

PATHOPHYSIOLOGY

There are a number of factors that affect wound healing and may cause a wound to fail to progress along the normal healing continuum. Factors that affect healing can be intrinsic or extrinsic, systemic or local.[3,5,7]

Age is considered an intrinsic factor that affects healing. There are a number of changes that occur with normal aging of the skin that may impede healing after injury. From a structural perspective the epidermis exhibits a flattening of the epidermal-dermal junction, changes in the basal cells, and a decrease in the number of Langerhans' cells and melanocytes.[2,4] This creates the following potential functional concerns:

♦ Altered skin permeability
♦ A decrease in inflammatory responsiveness
♦ A decrease in immunologic response
♦ Impaired wound healing

Changes in the dermal layer include a decrease in dermal thickness, a degeneration of elastin fibers, and a decrease in vascularization.[2,4] These changes that occur with normal aging will have functional implications, such as decreased elasticity, decrease in overall durability, slow wound healing, less scar tissue formation, and a decrease in vitamin D production. The dermal appendages are also affected through the normal aging process. The number of sweat glands and hair follicles decrease, resulting in a decrease in eccrine sweating and potential alteration in skin thermoregulation. The decrease in dermal appendages also impacts the potential to heal partial-thickness injuries that need new epithelial growth for resurfacing.[2]

Various factors that affect healing will be addressed in subsequent chapters and in several of the case studies. They will briefly be discussed here. A number of disease processes and co-morbidities have the potential to impair healing once injury occurs. Diseases that decrease the ability of oxygen and nutrients to reach injured areas are of particular concern. The presence of adequate blood supply and perfusion is essential for healing to occur. Diseases such as peripheral vascular disease (PVD), chronic anemia, and chronic obstructive pulmonary disease (COPD) will impede healing.[3,5,7]

Table 1-1	
LABORATORY VALUES OF NUTRITIONAL MARKERS	
Test (Blood)	Normal Range or Value
Albumin	3.5 to 5.5 g/dL
Prealbumin (adult)	15 to 43 mg/dL
Transferrin	200 to 400 mg/dL
Note: General guidelines, lab-dependent	

PVD, both arterial and venous, may impact wound healing or place a patient at risk for poor healing. Adequate vascularization and the importance of perfusion and oxygenation remain of utmost importance in wound healing.[3,5,7]

Diabetes, with its known damage to white blood cells and damage to the macrovascular system, is a significant risk factor to wound healing.[5]

Another intrinsic factor that may affect healing is immunosuppression, whether disease or medication induced. Immune suppression affects collagen synthesis during the proliferative phase, and the limited immune cells affect the inflammatory response phase.[7]

Malnutrition and dehydration also have a systemic effect on healing in that they may delay overall healing and also may be implicated in wound infections.[7] Protein is required for cellular repair. The need for increased amounts of protein should be considered when examining patients at risk for integumentary disruption and healing.[3,7] Laboratory values that provide information regarding nutritional status may be beneficial to assess the potential impact on healing or risk for integumentary disruption. Tests for nutritional status include albumin, prealbumin, and serum transferrin. Table 1-1 includes normal ranges of these nutritional markers.

Finally, from intrinsic and systemic perspectives, a patient who is obese has potential healing difficulties as a result of the increased stress on surgical incisions, the decrease in tissue perfusion, and the decrease in tissue oxygenation.[5]

A number of extrinsic factors are associated with risk of integumentary impairment. Certain medications are known for their detrimental effects on healing or on the tissues responsible for healing. Additional information on medications may be found in the Pharmacology section. Irradiation is another extrinsic factor. Radiation therapy is used to damage and kill cells. Radiation causes cellular injury to the fibroblasts, endothelial cells, and vascular supply in the area. Tissues that have undergone radiation will then be at risk for integumentary disruption and impaired healing.[7]

Stress has also been identified as an extrinsic factor associated with impaired healing. This appears to be in response to increased cortisol production and an ultimate decrease in the immune response.[5,7]

Bacterial burden or infection may be either systemic or local. Bacteria are present in most wounds, and it is the eventual bacterial burden that becomes infection. Infection is classified as a bacterial burden of greater than 10^5 organisms/gram of tissue.[12] One must recognize that bacteria are needed for wound healing and that granulation tissue is a normal response to an abnormal situation and requires some bacteria to be present in order to facilitate the neovascularization and repair process.[5]

Smoking is also an extrinsic factor that creates risk at a systemic level. Smoking causes vasoconstriction, an increase in platelet aggregation, and a decrease in available oxygen. All three of these factors will impede healing and place a patient at risk for integumentary disruption.[3]

Pressure on the skin is a considerable risk for certain patient populations and should be considered in any patient or client who has limited mobility. A pressure ulcer is a wound caused by unrelieved pressure against the skin over bony prominences. The result of pressure is local ischemia and potential tissue necrosis.[13]

Research is ongoing into those factors that may delay healing, impede healing, or place a patient at risk for integumentary disruption.

PHARMACOLOGY

Topical medications may include skin sealants to decrease the risk of urine and fecal contamination and moisture barriers to maintain skin hydration.

♦ Skin sealants and moisture barriers
  • Examples: Skin-Prep, SensiCare, 3M No Sting Skin Protectant
  • Actions: Form a protective layer or coating over the skin to prevent water, body fluids, or antimicrobial topical agents from irritating periwound tissue or as prevention to urine and fecal incontinence
  • Administered: Topically to the at-risk tissue
  • Side effects: Skin irritation
♦ Moisturizers
  • Examples: Over-the-counter petrolatum-based product
  • Actions: Effective at preventing and eliminating dry skin
  • Administered: Topically to at-risk areas
  • Side effects: Skin irritation

In addition, the following drugs that the client may be taking or may have taken may increase the risk of integumentary disruption.

♦ Glucocorticoids (corticosteroids, steroids)
  • Examples: Prednisone, cortisone, hydrocortisone
  • Side effects:
    ▪ Attenuates the inflammatory response
    ▪ Decreases vascular permeability

- Inhibits hypersensitivity reactions
- Has catabolic effect on bone, ligaments, tendons, and skin
  - Used for: Treatment of endocrine disorders and to resolve symptoms that are not endocrine related to include gastrointestinal disorders, respiratory conditions, and hypersensitivity reactions
- Antineoplastic medications
  - Examples: Fluorouracil, melphalan, dactinomycin, cisplatin
  - Side effects:
    - Blood disorders (anemia, leucopenia, thrombocytopenia)
    - Skin disorders
  - Used for: Treatment of cancers
- Immunosuppressive agents
  - Examples: Cyclosporine, azathioprine, sulfasalazine
  - Side effects:
    - Blood disorders
    - Skin disorders
    - Hypersensitivity reactions
  - Used for: Treatment of transplant rejection, rheumatoid arthritis (RA), multiple sclerosis (MS)

Case Study #1:
Integumentary Disruption Prevention

Mr. Timothy Brady is a 40-year-old male with a 10-year history of multiple sclerosis and is wheelchair bound.

PHYSICAL THERAPIST EXAMINATION

HISTORY

- General demographics: Mr. Brady is a 40-year-old white male whose primary language is English. He is left-hand dominant and is a college graduate.
- Social history: Mr. Brady is married and has two small dogs at home.
- Employment/work: He is a software engineer and is able to work from home while sitting for long hours in his electric wheelchair.
- Living environment: He resides in a wheelchair-accessible home.
- General health status
  - General health perception: Mr. Brady reports his health status as fair.
  - Physical function: He is severely limited requiring complete assistance for transfers into and out of his electric wheelchair. He is unable to perform pressure relief maneuvers.

- Psychological function: Normal.
- Role function: Husband, software engineer.
- Social function: He is limited in his ability to be out of the house secondary to issues of incontinence and the need for physical assistance with eating.
- Social/health habits: Mr. Brady does not smoke and rarely ingests alcohol.
- Family history: Noncontributory.
- Medical/surgical history: Mr. Brady has no significant past medical or surgical history other than his history of MS.
- Current condition(s)/chief complaint(s): He is seeking information regarding pressure relief and reassessment of his current electric wheelchair due to recent weight loss.
- Functional status and activity level: He is essentially totally dependent in all activities of daily living (ADL) and instrumental activities of daily living (IADL). He has set up his computer station to meet his limitations to include voice recognition systems so that he can work. He is able to use his electric wheelchair independently once transferred and positioned.
- Medications: Tylenol, Neurontin, Ditropan, heparin, Nizoral, and bacolofen.
- Other clinical tests
  - Lab values
    - Hemoglobin (Hgb)=11.8 g/dL (norm=14 to 16.5 g/dL)
    - Hematocrit (Hct)=35% (norm=42% to 52%)
    - Albumin=3.4 g/dL (norm=3.5 to 5.5 mg/dL)

SYSTEMS REVIEW

- Cardiovascular/pulmonary
  - Blood pressure (BP): 110/72 mmHg
  - Edema: None
  - Heart rate (HR): 68 bpm
  - Respiratory rate (RR): 12 rpm
- Integumentary
  - Presence of scar formation: None
  - Skin color: Within normal limits (WNL)
  - Skin integrity: WNL
- Musculoskeletal
  - Gross range of motion: Within functional limits (WFL)
  - Gross strength: Significantly limited
  - Gross symmetry: Asymmetrical
  - Height: 5'8" (1.727 m)
  - Weight: 140 lbs (63.5 kg)
- Neuromuscular
  - Balance: Unable to maintain unsupported sitting
  - Locomotion, transfers, and transitions: Requires complete assistance

Table 1-2
BODY MASS INDEX CATEGORIES

Numerical Score	Category
Below 18.5	Underweight
18.5 to 24.9	Normal
25.0 to 29.9	Overweight
30.0 and above	Obese

- Communication, affect, cognition, language, and learning style: WNL
  - Learning preferences: Visual learner

TESTS AND MEASURES

- Anthropometric characteristics
  - Body mass index (BMI): Weight (140 lbs, 63.5 kg) divided by height^2 (5'8", 1.727 m)=21.3 placing Mr. Brady at normal for his height and weight
  - Table 1-2 indicates BMI categories according to the Centers of Disease Control and Prevention[14]
- Circulation
  - Pulse exam: Revealed 2+ pulses bilaterally dorsalis pedis (DP) and posterior tibial (PT)
- Cranial and peripheral nerve integrity
  - Protective sensation
    - Semmes-Weinstein monofilament testing revealed intact protective sensation (see Table 4-5)
      - Monofilament testing is clinically useful in assessing normal light touch
      - Loss of protective sensation is classified as the inability to feel 10 grams of pressure utilizing a 5.07 monofilament[3]
- Environmental, home, and work barriers
  - Home environment is wheelchair accessible
- Ergonomics and body mechanics
  - Analysis of body mechanics while sitting in his wheelchair revealed:
    - Inability to alter body position for pressure relief
    - Inability to correct postural alignment once misalignment occurred
- Gait, locomotion, and balance
  - He required complete assistance for transfers in and out of his electric wheelchair
  - Once in his wheelchair he was able to maneuver the chair independently within his environment
- Integumentary integrity
  - Inspection and palpation revealed no evidence of infection, erythema, or edema
  - Risk assessment (eg, using Braden risk assessment tool)

- Braden risk assessment revealed 11/23 placing Mr. Brady at high risk
  - The Braden risk assessment tool appears to be the most widely used due to the amount of research on a variety of patient populations
  - It has also been shown to have the best validity and reliability[3,15-17]
  - The Braden Scale for Predicting Pressure Sore Risk consists of subscales that address mobility, activity, sensory perception, skin moisture, nutritional status, and friction and shear
  - Each subset is rated 1 to 4 except friction and shear that are rated 1 to 3
  - The overall score is between 6 and 23
  - A recent study indicated that a cutoff score of 18 was predictive of risk[3,11,13]
  - Table 1-3 describes the Braden Scale for Predicting Pressure Sore Risk[7]
  - Scores to identify risk include less than 12 indicates high risk, 13 to 15 moderate risk, and 16 to 18 mild risk
- Motor function
  - Unable to initiate motor control of his lower extremities (LEs)
  - Noted minimal antigravity movement of his upper extremities (UEs), left greater than right
- Muscle performance
  - Manual muscle testing was deferred secondary to significant motor function deficits
- Orthotic, protective, and supportive devices
  - Assessment of alignment and fit of wheelchair revealed good alignment and fit, but pressure relief cushion was in disrepair and did not allow for complete pressure relief of his right ischial tuberosity
- Pain
  - He reported general body pain of 3 out of 10 on a visual analog scale (VAS)
- Posture
  - Alignment and position: Deviation from midline
    - Mr. Brady required a lap belt and a slight posterior tilt of his wheelchair seat to assist with proper posture
    - He was unable to correct his posture if he became misaligned, requiring physical assistance periodically throughout the day
- Self-care and home management/work, community, and leisure integration or reintegration
  - Mr. Brady is totally dependent in self-care activities
  - During the interview, Mr. Brady reported occasional difficulty with fatigue, limiting his ability to work at his computer

- An additional area of concern was his increasing need for physical assistance and that his wife worked outside the home during the day

EVALUATION

Mr. Brady's history and risk factors previously outlined indicate that he is at high risk for pressure ulcer development. He also has significant deficits in motor control and physical functioning.

DIAGNOSIS

Mr. Brady is at risk for integumentary disruption. In addition, he has impaired: gait, locomotion, and balance; motor function; and muscle performance. He is functionally limited in self-care and home management and in work, community, and leisure actions, tasks, and activities. He is in need of orthotic, protective, and supportive devices. These findings are consistent with placement in Pattern A: Primary Prevention/Risk Reduction for Integumentary Disorders and in Neuromuscular Pattern E: Impaired Motor Function and Sensory Integrity Associated With Progressive Disorders of the Central Nervous System. These impairments and functional limitations will be addressed in determining the prognosis and the plan of care.

PROGNOSIS AND PLAN OF CARE

Over the course of the visits, the following mutually established outcomes have been determined:
- Ability to perform physical activities related to self-care and work is improved
- Knowledge of behaviors that foster healthy habits, wellness, and prevention is increased
- Level of assistance required for task performance is decreased
- Referrals are made to other professionals or resources
- Risk factors are reduced
- Tissue perfusion and oxygenation are enhanced

To achieve these outcomes, the appropriate interventions for this client are determined. These will include: coordination, communication, and documentation; patient/client-related instruction; therapeutic exercise; functional training in self-care and home management; functional training in work, community, and leisure integration or reintegration; and prescription, application, and, as appropriate, fabrication of devices and equipment.

Based on the diagnosis and prognosis, Mr. Brady is expected to require three to six visits over a 3-week period of time. Mr. Brady lives with his wife who works outside of the home, is motivated, and follows through with his home program. He is severely impaired, but generally healthy.

Table 1-3

BRADEN SCALE FOR PREDICTING PRESSURE SORE RISK

Sensory Perception Ability to respond to pressure-related stimuli	1. Completely limited 2. Very limited 3. Slightly limited 4. No impairment
Moisture Degree to which skin is exposed to moisture	1. Constantly moist 2. Very moist 3. Occasionally moist 4. Rarely moist
Activity Degree of physical activity	1. Bedfast 2. Chairfast 3. Walks occasionally 4. Walks frequently
Mobility Ability to alter and control body position	1. Completely immobile 2. Very limited 3. Slightly limited 4. No limitation
Nutrition Usual food intake	1. Very poor 2. Probably inadequate 3. Adequate 4. Excellent
Friction and Shear	1. Problem 2. Potential problem 3. No apparent problem

Adapted from Sussman C, Bates-Jensen BM, eds. *Wound Care: A Collaborative Practice Manual for Physical Therapists and Nurses.* Gaithersburg, Md: Aspen Publishers, Inc; 1998.

INTERVENTIONS

RATIONALE FOR SELECTED INTERVENTIONS

Pressure ulcers are a serious health care problem affecting patients across all care settings. Prevalence studies have seen rates as high as 15% in acute care hospitals[18] and 20% in nursing homes.[19] These numbers are likely to increase as the overall acuity of patients in the various settings continues to increase.[20] The cost of pressure ulcers to the health care system can be upwards of $40,000 per ulcer.[3] Prevention and early intervention can decrease morbidity and mortality associated with pressure ulcers, and the earlier interventions are initiated the better the potential outcome.[21]

COORDINATION, COMMUNICATION, AND DOCUMENTATION

Communication will occur with Mr. Brady and his primary caregiver, his wife. Additional referrals will be made to a nutritionist secondary to his recent weight loss. Ongoing communication will continue with his primary care physician. Additional referrals to address Mr. Brady's wheelchair and wheelchair cushion will also be made. All elements of the client's management will be documented.

PATIENT/CLIENT-RELATED INSTRUCTION

The client will be instructed in the risk factors related to pressure ulcers, the importance of positioning and pressure relief strategies, the importance of exercise to minimize secondary impairments, and the proper use of pressure relief devices. Particular emphasis will be related to education regarding pressure ulcer risk factors. Mr. Brady's wife and other family or friends, who may be assisting in his care, will be included in the education.

Mr. Brady and his family will be instructed in pressure relief strategies. Since Mr. Brady is a visual learner, education will be provided by demonstration and through on-line educational resources that pertain to pressure ulcer prevention.

THERAPEUTIC EXERCISE

♦ Body mechanics and postural stabilization
  ● Postural awareness training using visual feedback from a floor-length mirror
  ● Use of the tilt features of the wheelchair to assist with realignment
  ● Instruction to reassess postural alignment at least once an hour when working at the computer
♦ Flexibility exercises
  ● Passive range of motion (PROM) exercises to be taught to the client's wife and other family members

FUNCTIONAL TRAINING IN SELF-CARE AND HOME MANAGEMENT

♦ Self-care and home management
  ● Caregiver instruction will be given regarding injury prevention during transfers
  ● Caregiver will be instructed in provision of exercise programs

FUNCTIONAL TRAINING IN WORK, COMMUNITY, AND LEISURE INTEGRATION OR REINTEGRATION

♦ Work and community
  ● Injury prevention or reduction with use of devices and equipment

● Specific training in use of a new wheelchair cushion
● Specific training in the use of the reclining/elevating functions of client's electric wheelchair
● Use of appropriate incontinence management techniques will be reviewed

PRESCRIPTION, APPLICATION, AND, AS APPROPRIATE, FABRICATION OF DEVICES AND EQUIPMENT

♦ Protective devices
  ● Seating system will be reevaluated
  ● Pressure relief cushion will be obtained

ANTICIPATED GOALS AND EXPECTED OUTCOMES

♦ Impact on pathology/pathophysiology
  ● Tissue perfusion and oxygenation are enhanced by evidence of intact capillary refill.
♦ Impact on impairments
  ● Postural control is improved to be able to maintain positions for 15 minutes.
♦ Impact on functional limitations
  ● Ability to perform physical actions, tasks, and activities is improved with least amount of caregiver assistance.
  ● Ability to perform physical actions, tasks, and activities related to work, community, and leisure integration or reintegration is improved.
  ● Caregiver ability to perform physical actions, tasks, or activities related to self-care and home management is improved to independence in five visits.
  ● Tolerance of positions and activities is increased to be able to perform computer activities.
♦ Risk reduction/prevention
  ● Pressure on body tissues is reduced via positioning techniques, positioning devices, and pressure-reducing devices.
  ● Risk factors are reduced.
  ● Risk of secondary impairments is reduced.
  ● Self-management of symptoms is improved.
♦ Impact on health, wellness, and fitness
  ● Behaviors that foster healthy habits, wellness, and prevention are acquired.
  ● Health status is improved.
  ● Physical function is improved.
  ● Safety is improved.
♦ Impact on societal resources
  ● Documentation occurs throughout client management and follows APTA's *Guidelines for Physical Therapy Documentation*.[22]

- Referrals are made to other professionals or resources whenever necessary and appropriate, to include a nutritionist and wheelchair seating specialist.
  - Resources are utilized in a cost-effective way.
- Patient/client satisfaction
  - Client and family knowledge and awareness of the diagnosis, prognosis, interventions, and anticipated goals and outcomes are increased.
  - Sense of well-being and control is improved.

REEXAMINATION

Reexamination is performed throughout the episode of care.

DISCHARGE

Mr. Brady is discharged from physical therapy after a total of five physical therapy sessions and attainment of his goals and expectations. These sessions have covered his entire episode of care. He is discharged because he has achieved his goals and expected outcomes.

Case Study #2:
Integumentary Disruption Prevention

Mrs. Doris Smith is an 88-year-old female status post right femur fracture, currently in traction awaiting surgical fixation/repair.

PHYSICAL THERAPIST EXAMINATION

HISTORY

- General demographics: Mrs. Smith is an 88-year-old black American female whose primary language is English. She is right-hand dominant and is a college graduate.
- Social history: Mrs. Smith is widowed and has three children living in the area.
- Employment/work: She is retired but still participates in church activities regularly.
- Living environment: She resides in an assisted living facility.
- General health status
  - General health perception: Mrs. Smith reports that her health status is good.
  - Physical function: Prior to her recent fall and femoral

fracture, she was independently ambulating with a cane.
  - Psychological function: Normal.
  - Role function: Mother, grandmother, active church participant.
  - Social function: She was able to attend church regularly and participate in weekly church activities. She utilized the van from the assisted living facility to get to church, the grocery store, and to appointments.
- Social/health habits: Mrs. Smith does not smoke or ingest alcohol.
- Family history: Her mother died of heart disease and diabetes.
- Medical/surgical history: She has a history of osteoarthritis (OA) in her left hip and knee, hypertension (HTN), insulin dependent diabetes mellitus (IDDM), and peripheral artery disease (PAD).
- Current condition(s)/chief complaint(s): Mrs. Smith and her physician were seeking information regarding prevention from integumentary disruption while she awaited surgical repair of her right femoral fracture.
- Functional status and activity level: She is currently on complete bed rest with skeletal traction in place for her right femoral fracture.
- Medications: Lisinopril, insulin, Demerol via patient-controlled anesthesia (PCA) pump.
- Other clinical tests
  - Lab values
    - Hgb=13 g/dL (norm=12 to 15 g/dL)
    - Hct=40% (norm=35% to 47%)
    - Albumin=3.0 g/dL (norm=3.5 to 5.5 mg/dL)
  - Imaging studies
    - Fractures can be classified by location (proximal third, middle third, distal third), by the geometry of the fracture, or by the displacement, alignment, and comminution. A universal classification system for fractures does not exist. Two of the most common classification systems are the Winquist-Hansen[23] and Arbeitsgemeinschaft für osteosynthesefragen/Association for the Study of Internal Fixation (AO/ASIF) systems.[24]
    - Plain films revealed a Grade II femur fracture according to the Winquist-Hansen classification system that uses five categories.
      - 0=No comminution, simple transverse or oblique
      - I=Small butterfly fragment, minimal to no comminution
      - II=Butterfly fragment with at least 50% of the circumference of the cortices of the two major fragments intact
      - III=Butterfly fragment with 50% to 100% of

the circumference of the two major fragments comminuted

▸ IV=Segmental comminution, all cortical contact is lost[23]

SYSTEMS REVIEW

♦ Cardiovascular/pulmonary
  ● BP: 134/96 mmHg
  ● Edema: Moderate edema noted right foot
  ● HR: 72 bpm
  ● RR: 12 rpm
♦ Integumentary
  ● Presence of scar formation: None
  ● Skin color: WNL
  ● Skin integrity: WNL for observed area, unable to assess right lower extremity (RLE) secondary to traction set-up
♦ Musculoskeletal
  ● Gross range of motion: WFL except RLE deferred secondary to traction
  ● Gross strength: UEs and left lower extremity (LLE) were WFL, RLE deferred as noted above
  ● Gross symmetry: Symmetrical
  ● Height: 5'3" (1.6 m)
  ● Weight: 110 lbs (49.9 kg)
♦ Neuromuscular
  ● Balance: Unable to be assessed
  ● Locomotion, transfers, and transitions: Currently on complete bed rest
♦ Communication, affect, cognition, language, and learning style: WNL
  ● Learning preferences: Visual learner

TESTS AND MEASURES

♦ Anthropometric characteristics
  ● BMI: Weight (110 lbs, 49.9 kg) divided by height^2 (5'3", 1.6 m)=19.5 BMI placing Mrs. Smith in the normal category
♦ Circulation
  ● Pulse exam: Revealed 1+ pulses on the left DP and PT and 2+ on the right DP and PT
♦ Cranial and peripheral nerve integrity
  ● Protective sensation
    ■ Semmes-Weinstein monofilament testing revealed intact protective sensation (see Table 4-5)
♦ Integumentary integrity
  ● Inspection and palpation revealed no evidence of infection or erythema
  ● Edema: 1+ pitting edema noted on the dorsum of the right foot

● Risk assessment (eg, using the Braden scale)
  ■ Braden risk assessment tool revealed 16/23 placing Mrs. Smith at minimum risk
  ■ See information from Case Study #1 regarding risk assessment tools for pressure ulcers
♦ Orthotic, protective, and supportive devices
  ● Traction set-up appears to be intact with good contact and padding to minimize pressure
♦ Pain
  ● 5 out of 10 in RLE at traction pin sites on a VAS
♦ Self-care and home management
  ● Mrs. Smith is able to perform her upper body ADL independently, such as eating and grooming
  ● She requires assistance with rolling and turning secondary to her traction set-up

EVALUATION

Mrs. Smith's history and risk factors previously outlined indicate that she is at minimum risk for pressure ulcer development. Mrs. Smith will need additional therapy examination and interventions once she undergoes surgical correction of her femur fracture.

DIAGNOSIS

Mrs. Smith has sustained a right femoral fracture and has pain at the pin sites. She has impaired circulation and integumentary integrity. She is functionally limited in self-care actions, tasks, and activities. She is at risk for integumentary disruption placing her in Pattern A: Primary Prevention/Risk Reduction for Integumentary Disorders. These impairments and functional limitations will be addressed in determining the prognosis and the plan of care.

PROGNOSIS AND PLAN OF CARE

Over the course of the visits, the following mutually established outcomes have been determined:
♦ Knowledge of behaviors that foster healthy habits, wellness, and prevention is increased
♦ Referrals are made to other professionals or resources

To achieve these outcomes, the appropriate interventions for this client are determined. These will include: coordination, communication, and documentation; patient/client-related instruction; therapeutic exercise; and functional training in self-care and home management.

Mrs. Smith is expected to require one to three visits. Mrs. Smith has good social support and is motivated. She is impaired, but otherwise healthy.

INTERVENTIONS

Rationale for selected interventions can be found in Case Study #1 and in Musculoskeletal Pattern A: Primary Prevention/Risk Reduction for Skeletal Demineralization.

COORDINATION, COMMUNICATION, AND DOCUMENTATION

Communication will occur with Mrs. Smith's primary care physician. She will be referred to the nutrition service secondary to a slightly lower than normal albumin level. All elements of the client's management will be documented.

PATIENT/CLIENT-RELATED INSTRUCTION

The client and family will be instructed in the risk factors related to potential integumentary disruption and pressure ulcer prevention. Mrs. Smith will be instructed in the performance of pressure-relieving movements within the confines of her hospital bed and will ask for assistance in turning. She will be instructed in the importance of maintaining adequate nutrition and hydration.

THERAPEUTIC EXERCISE

- Body mechanics and postural stabilization
  - The client will be assisted in postural awareness in relation to the need for pressure relief
- Flexibility exercises
  - General range of motion (ROM) exercises of both UEs and LLE to maintain flexibility
- Strength, power, and endurance training
  - UE weight training with elastic bands
  - Breathing exercises to enhance oxygen exchange and prevent pulmonary complications

FUNCTIONAL TRAINING IN SELF-CARE AND HOME MANAGEMENT

- Injury prevention or reduction
  - Education regarding risk factors while performing functional activities in her hospital bed
  - Education in the traction set-up to allow for pressure relief
  - Education in the signs and symptoms of pressure

ANTICIPATED GOALS AND EXPECTED OUTCOMES

- Impact on pathology/pathophysiology
  - Tissue perfusion and oxygenation are enhanced by evidence of intact capillary refill.
- Impact on impairments
  - Sensory awareness is increased.

- Impact on functional limitations
  - Ability to perform physical actions, tasks, or activities related to self-care is improved while she remains in skeletal traction.
  - Pain is decreased to 2/10 while performing self-care activities.
- Risk reduction/prevention
  - Risk factors are reduced with respect to pressure ulcer prevention.
  - Risk of secondary impairments is reduced.
- Impact on health, wellness, and fitness
  - Physical function is improved within the confines of skeletal traction.
- Impact on societal resources
  - Documentation occurs throughout client management and follows APTA's *Guidelines for Physical Therapy Documentation*.[22]
  - Intensity of care is decreased.
  - Referrals are made to other professionals or resources whenever necessary and appropriate to include a nutrition referral.
  - Resources are utilized in a cost-effective way.
  - Utilization of physical therapy services is optimized.
- Patient/client satisfaction
  - Client and family knowledge and awareness of the diagnosis, prognosis, interventions, and anticipated goals and outcomes are increased.
  - Client understanding of anticipated goals and expected outcomes is increased.
  - Sense of well-being is enhanced.

REEXAMINATION

Reexamination is performed throughout the episode of care.

DISCHARGE

Mrs. Smith is discharged from physical therapy for prevention of integumentary disruption after a total of two physical therapy sessions and attainment of her goals and expectations. These sessions have covered her entire episode of care. She is discharged from this phase of her interventions because she has achieved her goals and expected outcomes.

Case Study #3:
Integumentary Disruption Prevention

Ms. Amy O'Shea is a 38-year-old female with a new diagnosis of rheumatoid arthritis.

PHYSICAL THERAPIST EXAMINATION

HISTORY

♦ General demographics: Ms. O'Shea is a 38-year-old white female whose primary language is English. She is right-hand dominant and is a currently pursuing a college degree part-time.

♦ Social history: Ms. O'Shea is divorced and has no children.

♦ Employment/work: She is employed as an administrative assistant. She attends a university part-time and is active within her community.

♦ Living environment: She resides in a single-story home with stairs to enter.

♦ General health status
  • General health perception: Ms. O'Shea reports that her health status is good.
  • Physical function: Her reported physical function is normal for her age.
  • Psychological function: Normal.
  • Role function: Daughter, administrative assistant, student.
  • Social function: She works full-time, attends school two evenings a week, and participates regularly in the local soup kitchen as a volunteer.

♦ Social/health habits: Ms. O'Shea does not smoke and drinks wine occasionally.

♦ Family history: She has an aunt with RA.

♦ Medical/surgical history: Ms. O'Shea has no other significant history.

♦ Current condition(s)/chief complaint(s): Ms. O'Shea has just been recently diagnosed with RA. The diagnostic criteria for RA, established by the American Rheumatism Association includes: 1) morning stiffness for at least 6 weeks, 2) inflammatory changes in three or more joints for at least 6 weeks, 3) swelling in the wrist or metacarpal joints for at least 6 weeks, 4) symmetrical joint swelling, 5) radiographic evidence, 6) nodules, and/or 7) a positive rheumatoid factor blood test. Patients must have four or more of the seven conditions listed above to be diagnosed with RA.[2] On the advice of her physician, Ms. O'Shea was seeking information regarding prevention of integumentary disruption secondary to steroid use, prevention of osteoporosis (see

Musculoskeletal Pattern A: Primary Prevention/Risk Reduction for Skeletal Demineralization), and an exercise program to maintain her current level of fitness.

♦ Functional status and activity level: She is independent in all ADL and IADL. She indicates that she generally exercises at least three times a week swimming or walking.

♦ Medications: Disease-modifying antirheumatic drugs (DMARDs), prednisone, nonsteroidal anti-inflammatory drugs (NSAIDs), a multivitamin, and calcium supplement

♦ Other clinical tests
  • Lab values
    ▪ Hgb=15 g/dL
    ▪ Hct=40%
    ▪ Erythrocyte sedimentation rate (ESR)=110 mm/hr (normal: <30 to 40 mm/hr)
    ▪ Rheumatoid factor: Positive
      ‣ Rheumatoid factor is not necessarily an indicator that someone in fact has RA, because it can also be seen in the normal population[2]
    ▪ C-reactive protein: Normal
      ‣ C-reactive protein is an indicator of systemic inflammation and is used as a predictor of disease outcome in the RA population[2]
  • Radiographic films revealed mild periarticular swelling and cortical thinning on the left wrist as compared to the right

SYSTEMS REVIEW

♦ Cardiovascular/pulmonary
  • BP: 118/72 mmHg
  • Edema: Minimal digital swelling noted
  • HR: 64 bpm
  • RR: 10 rpm

♦ Integumentary
  • Presence of scar formation: None
  • Skin color: WNL
  • Skin integrity: WNL

♦ Musculoskeletal
  • Gross range of motion: WFL
  • Gross strength: WFL
  • Gross symmetry: Symmetrical
  • Height: 5'7" (1.7 m)
  • Weight: 140 lbs (63.5 kg)

♦ Neuromuscular
  • Balance: No unsteadiness observed
  • Locomotion, transfers, and transitions: WNL

♦ Communication, affect, cognition, language, and learning style: WNL

- Expected emotional/behavioral responses: Eager to have information regarding prevention and risk factor modifications
- Learning preferences: Visual learner

TESTS AND MEASURES

- Aerobic capacity/endurance
  - 1-Mile Walk test=12.5 minutes (excellent for client's age). The 1-Mile Walk test for women between 30 to 39 years has the following categories: excellent=less than 13:42 minutes, good=13:42 to 14:36 minutes, average=14:37 to 15:36 minutes, fair=15:37 to 17:00 minutes, and poor=greater than 17 minutes[25]
- Anthropometric characteristics
  - BMI: Weight (140 lbs, 63.5 kg) divided by height^2 (5'7", 1.7 m)=21.9 BMI placing her in the normal category
- Arousal, attention, and cognition
  - Outcome Expectations for Exercise (OEE) indicated awareness of exercise benefits
- Circulation
  - Pulse exam: Revealed 2+ pulses bilaterally DP and PT
- Environmental, home, and work barriers: None
- Gait, locomotion, and balance
  - One-Legged Stance test revealed ability to maintain one-legged stance with eyes closed for at least 30 seconds on both LEs
  - Gait observed was normal without deviations
- Integumentary integrity
  - Inspection and palpation revealed no evidence of infection, erythema, or edema
  - Risk assessment (eg, using the Braden scale)
    - Braden risk assessment tool revealed 23/23 placing Ms. O'Shea at no risk for pressure ulcer formation
    - See information from Case Study #1 regarding risk assessment tools for pressure ulcers
- Muscle performance
  - Manual muscle testing revealed 5/5 strength throughout with complaints of mild discomfort with grasp testing
- Pain
  - 3 out of 10 on a VAS during test of grasp bilaterally
- Posture
  - Observational assessment revealed
    - Slight forward head
- Range of motion
  - WFL throughout except decrease noted in full grasp, unable to approximate digital tips to distal palmar crease

- Self-care and home management/work, community, and leisure integration or reintegration
  - Ms. O'Shea indicated no difficulty with self-care, home management, work, community, or leisure activities as long as she maintained her medication regime

EVALUATION

Ms. O'Shea's history and risk factors previously outlined indicate that she is at no risk for pressure ulcer development, but due to corticosteroid use, she may be at risk for integumentary disruption and skeletal demineralization (see Musculoskeletal Pattern A: Primary Prevention/Risk Reduction for Skeletal Demineralization for additional information).

DIAGNOSIS

Ms. O'Shea has been recently diagnosed with RA with pain during grasp. She is at risk for integumentary disruption. These findings are consistent with placement in Pattern A: Primary Prevention/Risk Reduction for Integumentary Disorders. This risk will be addressed in determining the prognosis and the plan of care.

PROGNOSIS AND PLAN OF CARE

Over the course of the visits, the following mutually established outcomes have been determined:
- Ability to perform physical activities related to self-care and work is improved
- Knowledge of behaviors that foster healthy habits, wellness, and prevention is increased
- Risk factors (decreased physical activity, ROM, integumentary disruption) are reduced
- Risk of secondary impairments (integumentary disruption, fracture) are reduced

To achieve these outcomes, the appropriate interventions for this client are determined. These will include: coordination, communication, and documentation; patient/client-related instruction; and therapeutic exercise.

Based on the diagnosis and prognosis, Ms. O'Shea is expected to require between two to four visits over a 2-week period of time. Ms. O'Shea is motivated and will follow through with her home program. She is not severely impaired and is generally healthy.

INTERVENTIONS

Rationale for selected interventions can be found in Case Study #1 and in Pattern A: Primary Prevention/Risk Reduction for Skeletal Demineralization.

COORDINATION, COMMUNICATION, AND DOCUMENTATION

All elements of the client's management will be documented. A referral to a nutritionist will be made to ensure an appropriate diet secondary to her risk for integumentary and skeletal impairments.

PATIENT/CLIENT-RELATED INSTRUCTION

The client will be instructed regarding the risk factors for integumentary disruption and skeletal demineralization as a result of her need for long-term corticosteroid use. Ms. O'Shea will also be referred to a nutritionist to maximize her nutritional status.

THERAPEUTIC EXERCISE

♦ Aerobic capacity/endurance conditioning
  • Parameters for aerobic capacity/endurance conditioning or reconditioning (see Musculoskeletal Pattern A: Primary Prevention/Risk Reduction for Skeletal Demineralization)
♦ Relaxation
  • Complementary exercise approaches
    ▪ General relaxation exercises and techniques
    ▪ Ms. O'Shea was encouraged to participate in a regular relaxation program that may include Yoga
♦ Strength, power, and endurance training
  • Progressive stretching exercises
  • Review and modification of current exercise regime to increase weightbearing exercises

ANTICIPATED GOALS AND EXPECTED OUTCOMES

♦ Impact on functional limitations
  • Pain is decreased to 1/10 during grasp activities.
♦ Risk reduction/prevention
  • Risk factors are reduced.
  • Risk of secondary impairments is reduced.
♦ Impact on health, wellness, and fitness
  • Behaviors that foster healthy habits, wellness, and prevention are acquired.
  • Health status is improved.
♦ Impact on societal resources
  • Documentation occurs throughout client management and follows APTA's Guidelines for Physical Therapy Documentation.[22]
  • Referrals are made to other professionals or resources whenever necessary and appropriate.
  • Resources are utilized in a cost-effective way.
♦ Patient/client satisfaction

• Client knowledge and awareness of the diagnosis, prognosis, interventions, and anticipated goals and expected outcomes are increased.
• Client understanding of anticipated goals and expected outcomes is increased.
• Sense of well-being is improved.

REEXAMINATION

Reexamination is performed throughout the episode of care.

DISCHARGE

Ms. O'Shea is discharged from physical therapy after a total of three visits and attainment of her goals and expectations. These sessions have covered her entire episode of care. She is discharged because she has achieved her goals and expected outcomes.

REFERENCES

1. Corwin EJ. Handbook of Pathophysiology. 2nd ed. Philadelphia, Pa: Lippincott; 2000.
2. Goodman CC, Boissonnault WG, Fuller KS. Pathology Implications for the Physical Therapist. Philadelphia, Pa: Saunders; 2003.
3. Myers BA. Wound Management Principles and Practice. Upper Saddle River, NJ: Prentice Hall; 2004.
4. McCance KL, Huether SE. Pathophysiology: The Biologic Basis for Disease in Adults & Children. 4th ed. Philadelphia, Pa: Mosby; 2002.
5. Kloth LC, McCulloch JM. Wound Healing Alternatives in Management. 3rd ed. Philadelphia, Pa: FA Davis Co; 2002.
6. Histology. http://www3.umdnj.edu/histsweb/lab11/lab11thinskin/html. Accessed August 9, 2004.
7. Sussman C, Bates-Jensen BM, eds. Wound Care: A Collaborative Practice Manual for Physical Therapists and Nurses. Gaithersburg, Md: Aspen Publishers, Inc; 1998.
8. Kucan JO, Brown R, Hickerson W, et al. Plastic and Reconstructive Surgery Essential for Students. Arlington Heights, Ill: Plastic Surgery Educational Foundation; 1993.
9. Schultz GS. Wound bed preparation: a systematic approach to wound management. Wound Repair Regen. 2003;11(2 Suppl): S1-S28.
10. Lazarus GS. Definitions and guidelines for assessment of wound and evaluation of healing. Wound Repair Regen. 1994;2(3):165-170.
11. Falanga V. Wound bed preparation: future approaches. European Pressure Ulcer Advisory Panel Meeting, held in Budapest on September 19, 2002. Ostomy/Wound Management. 2003;49(5A Suppl):30-36.
12. Robson MC. Wound infection in the surgical patient: an imbalance in the normal equilibrium. Clin Plast Surg. 1979;6:493.
13. Bergstrom N, Bennett MA, Carlson CE, et al. Treatment of

Pressure Ulcers: Clinical Practice Guideline No. 15. Rockville, Md: US Department of Health and Human Services, Agency for Health Care Policy and Research; 1994.

14. BMI: body mass index. http://wwwcdc.gov/nccdphp/dnpa/bmi/calc-bmi.htm. Accessed September 1, 2004.

15. Bergstrom N, Braden BJ, Kemp MG, Champagne M, Ruby E. Predicting pressure ulcer risk: a multi-site study of the predictive validity of the Braden scale. *Nurs Res.* 1998;47(5):261-269.

16. Bergstrom N, Demuth PJ, Braden BJ. A clinical trial of the Braden scale for predicting pressure sore risk. *Nurs Clin North Am.* 1987;22(2):417-428.

17. Braden BJ, Bergstrom N. Clinical utility for the Braden scale for predicting pressure ulcers. *Decubitis.* 1989;2(3):45-51.

18. Amlung SR, Miller WL, Bosley LM. The 1999 national pressure ulcer prevalence survey: a bench-marking approach. *Advances in Skin and Wound Care.* 2001;14(6):297-301.

19. Kanj LF, Wilking SVB, Phillips TJ. Pressure ulcers. *J Am Acad Dermatol.* 1998;38(4):517-536.

20. Bennett RG, O'Sullivan J, Devito EM, Remsburg R. The increasing medical malpractice risk related to pressure ulcers in the United States. *J Am Geriatr Soc.* 2000;48:73-81.

21. Bergstrom N, Bennett MA, Carlson CE, et al. *Pressure Ulcers: Prevalence and Prevention Clinical Practice Guideline No. 3.* Rockville, Md: US Department of Health and Human Services, Agency for Health Care Policy and Research; 1992.

22. American Physical Therapy Association. Guide to physical therapist practice. 2nd ed. *Phys Ther.* 2001;81:9-744.

23. Wastwood B, Biggs HK, Knutson T. Diaphyseal femur fracture. *Emedicine.* Online article found at: http://wwwemedicine.com/orthoped/topic71.htm. Accessed September 6, 2004.

24. Wong KL, Williams GR. Proximal humeral fractures: diagnosis and management. *University of Pennsylvania Orthopaedic Journal.* Online article found at: http://www.uphs.upenn.edu/ortho/oj/1998/0j11sp98p1.html. Accessed December 28, 2004.

25. Mile walk test. Online article found at: http://www.walkwithremar.com/counch%20one-mile%test.htm. Accessed September 11, 2004.

CHAPTER TWO

Impaired Integumentary Integrity Associated With Superficial Skin Involvement (Pattern B)

Carrie Sussman, PT, DPT

ANATOMY

The skin, the largest organ in the body, has a layered structure. The outermost layer of the skin is called the epidermis or stratum corneum. The stratum corneum is an avascular structure that functions as a barrier to the environment and prevents transepidermal water loss.[1] Recent studies demonstrate that enzymatic activity is involved in the formation of an acid mantle in the stratum corneum. Together the acid mantle and the stratum corneum make the skin less permeable to water and other polar compounds, thereby indirectly protecting the skin from invasion by microorganisms. Normal surface skin pH is between 4 and 6.5 in healthy people but varies according to area of skin on the body. Damage of the stratum corneum is shown to increase skin pH and thus the susceptibility of the skin to bacterial skin infections.[2] For example, hand washing three times a day with cleansing agents alters the acid mantle for several hours. Multiple washings alter the barrier function including the skin pH for up to 14 hours with additional damage occurring with each subsequent washing. Diseases associated with increased skin surface pH include eczema, contact dermatitis, atopic dermatitis, and dry skin. Systemic diseases, including diabetes, chronic renal failure, and cerebrovascular disease, may also cause an increase in skin pH. Wound dressings and diapers have been known to raise the skin pH.[2]

Wound dressing adhesives are responsible for stripping the stratum corneum, causing noticeable transepidermal water loss.[1] The skin interprets this as a trauma and an inflammatory wound healing response is triggered that is proportional to the amount of damage to the skin. Skin cleansers and moisturizers that have low pH or neutral pH, in other words more alkaline, are suggested choices for maintaining the acid mantle of the skin. Soaps are more alkaline than most synthetic detergents and nonionic surfactants, which are slightly acidic or neutral, and thus may be the best choice to protect skin surface integrity.[2]

Other layers of the epidermis include: the stratum lucidum, stratum granulosum, stratum spinosum, and stratum germinativum (basale), all of which contain living cells. Melanin produced by melanocytes in the epidermis is responsible for the color of the skin. The immune processing cells, the Langerhans' cells, are also found in the epidermis. The epidermis relies entirely on the blood vessels in the dermis for nutrients. Dermal appendages include hair follicles, sebaceous glands, and sweat glands. Fingernails and toenails originate in the epidermis and protrude into the dermis.[3]

The basement membrane layer both separates and connects the epidermis and the dermis. When epidermal cells in the basement membrane divide, one cell stays there and the other migrates through the granular layer to the surface stratum corneum. At the surface, the cell dies and forms keratin on the skin surface.[3] The basement membrane atrophies with age, and separation between the basement membrane and the dermis is one cause for skin tears in the elderly.

The dermis is a vascular structure that supports and nourishes the epidermis. In addition, there are sensory nerve endings in the dermis that transmit signals regarding pain, pressure, heat, and cold. It may be divided into two layers: the superficial dermis and the deep dermis. The superficial dermis consists of collagen, elastin, and ground substances (ECM) and blood vessels. Fibroblasts are responsible for producing the collagen and elastin components of the skin that give it turgor. Fibronectin and hyaluronic acid are secreted by the fibroblasts. The deep dermis is located over the subcutaneous fat with a larger network of blood vessels and collagen fibers to provide tensile strength.[3]

PHYSIOLOGY/PATHOPHYSIOLOGY

EPIDERMAL WOUND HEALING

Closing the wound quickly and efficiently is a function of the epidermis. When the epidermis is injured, the body is subject to invasion by outside agents and loss of body fluids. Epidermal wounds heal primarily by cell migration. Clusters of epidermal cells migrate into the area of damage and cover the defect. These lead cells are phagocytic and clear the surface of debris and plasma clots. Winter[4] found that this cell migration progresses best in a moist environment. Repair cells originate from local sources that are primarily the dermal appendages and from adjacent intact skin areas. Healing occurs rapidly, and the skin is left unscarred.[4] Blisters are examples of epidermal wounds. They may be small vesicles or larger bullae (greater than 1 cm in diameter). Dry keratin on the surface is called scale. Hyperkeratosis, which is thickened layers of keratin, is often found on the heels and may be an indication of loss of sebaceous gland and sweat gland functions if the patient has diabetes.[5]

DERMAL WOUND HEALING

Dermal wounds involve the epidermis, basal membrane, and dermis. A dermal injury typically heals rapidly. Cracks in the dermis may exude serum, blood, or pus and may lead to formation of clots or crusts. Pustules are pus-filled vesicles that often represent infected hair follicles that are anchored in the dermis.

SKIN HYDRATION AND LUBRICATION

Moisture balance is important to maintain skin integrity. Extremes of dryness or hydration are equally damaging. Stratum corneum hydration and lubrication are important in keeping the skin intact. Halkier-Sorenson[6] has done extensive research on the barrier function of the stratum corneum. According to Halkier-Sorenson,[6] any disruption

in the stratum corneum will allow increased transepidermal water loss and almost complete secretion of lamellar body contents from the uppermost granular layer into the intercellular spaces of the stratum corneum impairing the barrier function. Normal adult skin has the capacity to recover its barrier function within 6 hours. During the recovery period there is an increase in lipid production within the stratum corneum.

Application of an effective moisturizer product with the appropriate mix of lipids can reduce the epidermal water loss during the recovery period. Oils and humectants are used to lubricate and hydrate the skin. Topical creams and ointments may assist in rehydration and lubrication but may also contain potential allergens.

Aged skin loses the capacity to recover in a normal fashion. Recovery of the barrier is slower. Barrier disruption causes a localized inflammatory cascade that is instrumental in the development of inflammatory skin diseases, such as eczema. Understanding the mechanisms and sites of action helps in selecting skin care products that restore barrier function. Theoretically, a moisturizer may affect the epidermis to varying depths. It may:

- Stay on the surface of the stratum corneum
- Penetrate into the intercellular spaces of the stratum corneum
- Penetrate into the viable epidermis and eventually become incorporated into the cells and later secreted

Early application of a skin barrier product will reduce transepidermal water loss and give the skin time to repair the stratum corneum. A good moisturizer can reduce the effect of the initial insult to the stratum corneum and block penetration of substances that may further injure the tissue. Petrolatum- and lanolin-based skin care products have been shown to enhance barrier recovery by reducing water loss and inhibiting the inflammatory reaction of the cells leading to a significant decrease in skin breakdown and pressure ulcers in elderly nursing home residents.[6,7]

INTRINSIC FACTORS ASSOCIATED WITH SUPERFICIAL INTEGUMENTARY IMPAIRMENTS

Age

Physiologic changes occur with aging and include:
- Slowed cell division, migration, and maturation[8]
- Increased metalloproteinases levels that are risk factors for integumentary breakdown[9]
- Loss of skin elasticity that in turn increases risk of injury to the integument
- Compromised circulatory, immune, and respiratory systems
- Altered hormonal responses that affect skin turgor

- Thinning of the skin
- Increased dryness
- Low surface humidity

Wound healing is delayed with aging because trauma to deep tissues is likely to cause internal bleeding due to changes in the capillary structure of the internal tissues, friability of the tissues, and blood thinning medications. Age is associated with chronic disease states that may be considered a marker for predisposition to skin breakdown.[10]

Chronic Disease States

Vascular Disease

Ischemia associated with atherosclerosis is indicated by changes in the integument. Atherosclerosis occurs earlier and more often in persons with diabetes. Clinical signs include a loss of hair and dry scaly skin due to loss of sebaceous and sweat glands. Additional clinical signs of ischemia include dependent rubor, pallor with elevation of the extremity, and intermittent claudication. Skin temperature, particularly of the distal extremities, may be cool or cold to touch. Individual toes may be dark or black.[11]

The clinical signs and symptoms of venous insufficiency include edema, varicose veins, pain, color changes in the integument, and dermatitis followed by ulceration.[12] Superficial skin changes that are associated with venous system disease include lipodermatosclerosis (the progressive hardening of the skin and subcutaneous tissue), hemosiderin staining, and edema that puts excess tension and internal pressure on the skin so that the skin may develop weeping.[13] Skin color is darkened in darkly pigmented skin and looks brown or brawny in lightly pigmented skin due to hemosiderin staining.

Edema is often the initial complaint that develops without warning and worsens during the day, especially after prolonged standing. At this stage, the edema resolves during the night. Venous edema is first seen at the ankle and then progresses proximally up to the knee. During the early stages, edema may pit, but if it is left unresolved, there are chronic changes of induration and fibrosis. At this stage the pitting disappears.[12] Dilated and tortuous veins at the medial side of the ankle accompanied by a sunburst of dilated small venular channels extending inferiorly from the medial malleolus may appear. This is referred to as "the ankle flare" sign and is considered pathognomonic of chronic venous insufficiency.[12] The patient's history may include trauma to the lower leg or history of deep vein thrombosis (DVT).

In 1996, a new classification of chronic venous disease (CVD) based on clinical, etiological, anatomic, and pathophysiolgic (CEAP) data was tested, and it was reported that this classification accurately identifies categories of CVD. The seven categories in descending order of severity are seen in Table 2-1. The assessment of the validity of the CEAP classification showed a good ascending severity but poorer

Table 2-1

CEAP CLASSIFICATION OF CHRONIC VENOUS DISEASE

Class	Definition
0	No visible or palpable signs of venous disease
1	Telangiectases or reticular veins
2	Varicose veins
3	Edema
4	Skin changes ascribed to venous disease (pigmentation, venous eczema, lipodermatosclerosis)
5	Skin changes (as defined above) in conjunction with healed ulcer
6	Skin changes (as defined above) in conjunction with active ulcer

CEAP=Clinical, etiologic, anatomic, pathophysiologic
From Kistner R, Eklof B, Masuda E. Diagnosis of chronic venous disease of the lower extremities: the "CEAP" classification. *Mayo Clin Proc*. 1996;71:338-345 with permission.

additivity.[14] The authors who reported this appraisal suggested that this basic tool would benefit from some refinements to make it better for clinical research of chronic venous disorders.[15]

Diabetic Polyneuropathies

Peripheral polyneuropathy associated with diabetes mellitus usually has a gradual onset that may include numbness, tingling, burning, and pins and needles. However, in some cases there is painful sudden onset of symptoms followed by sensory loss. Individuals with long-term diabetes, greater than 5 years of either Type 1 or 2 diabetes, show nervous system changes and may demonstrate one or up to three types of distal symmetric neuropathy referred to as polyneuropathy.[16]

Sensory Neuropathy

Sensory loss contributes to the loss of protective sensation of the extremities that usually occurs from distal to proximal and is progressive over time. Loss of protective sensation is considered a primary cause of skin ulceration in individuals and an indictor of risk for tissue ulceration. Testing for loss of protective sensation is done using Semmes-Weinstein monofilaments. The current standard test is to use a 10-gram (5.07 Semmes-Weinstein) nylon monofilament mounted on a holder that has been standardized to deliver a 10-gram force when properly applied to the surface of the skin. According to research findings, the ability to feel the 10-gram filament on at least two to five sites on the plantar surface of the foot (metatarsal heads and great toe) reduces the risk for ulceration.[16] Sensory loss also may mean that the individual does not have the ability to distinguish temperature variations,

Table 2-2	
WAGNER DYSVASCULAR SCALE	
Grade 0	A preulcerative lesion, healed ulcer, or presence of bony deformity
Grade 1	A superficial ulcer with subcutaneous tissue involvement
Grade 2	Penetration through the subcutaneous tissue and may have exposed bone, tendon, ligament, or joint capsule
Grade 3	Osteitis, abscess, or osteomyelitis

Adapted from Wagner FEW. The dysvascular foot: a system for diagnosis and treatment. *Foot and Ankle.* 1981;(2):64-122.

both hot and cold, which can result in superficial injury to the skin in the form of first-degree burns or frostbite. Tests for thermal sensitivity are performed by placing glass vials with warm or cold water against the side of the foot and noting the individual's response.[17]

Vibratory Sensation

Vibratory sensation is tested qualitatively by placing a 128-Hz tuning fork to the tip of the hallux and bony prominences. Either the vibration is felt or not. For a semiquantitative measure of vibratory perception threshold, an electronic tuning fork is suggested. Signals vary from 10 to 50 Hz. Checking vibratory sensation at regular intervals may be used to quantify sensory loss and loss of nerve function over time. Decreases in vibratory sensation are highly predictive of foot ulceration.[18]

Motor Neuropathy

Motor neuropathy contributes to muscular atrophy and change in alignment of the bony structures of the foot contributing to anatomic deformities. This has been called the "intrinsic minus foot."[19] Motor loss of the intrinsic muscles (lumbricales and interossei) results in claw toes progressing to foot drop. Involvement typically starts at the base of the first and fifth toes and progresses to all toes. As the muscles denervate, muscular imbalance occurs between the flexors and extensors resulting in flexion of the interphalangeal (IP) joints and extension at the metatarsophalangeal (MTP) joints and are referred to as hammer toes or claw foot deformity. The extension of the MTP joints causes the appearance of sharp bony prominences at the base of the toes resulting in areas of high pressure. Visible muscular atrophy accompanies these changes. As the sequelae of events continue, the extension of the MTP joints will eventually force upward rotation (supination) of the entire forefoot. The extensor hallucis longus is often affected by imbalance leading to hyperextension of the great toe with a prominent extensor tendon called a "cock-up" deformity.[19] The prominent metatarsal heads during weightbearing push the metatarsal fat pad distally, so it no longer provides cushioning over these areas of high

pressures. Callus will often appear in these areas.[19,20] These deformities increase the risk for injury and increase the healing times after injury has occurred.[21]

Autonomic neuropathy is the loss of sweat and sebaceous gland function leaving the skin dry and non-elastic, progressing to xerosis and hyperkeratosis.[17] Loss of sweat and sebaceous gland function predisposes the skin to changes in pH resulting in loss of the natural flora on the skin surface, making the skin more susceptible to infection.[5]

Circulatory Changes Associated With Diabetes

Diabetes affects the circulatory system resulting in calcification of the arterial walls of the distal vessels and restriction of local blood flow to the feet. Additionally, circulatory problems including the development of occlusive arterial disease below the knee may also occur. Blockages at the lower calf level may go undetected due to diabetic neuropathy. These blockages are often associated with low ankle artery BPs. The lower arterial perfusion to the digits of the feet may not be identified until after injury or gangrene develops.[22]

Venous disease in persons with diabetes is related to the loss of autonomic nervous system function. Physiologically, the arterial pulse acts on the deep leg veins to propel the blood back toward the heart. When atherosclerosis develops, the arterial vessels stiffen and alter blood propulsion. Motor neuropathy of the muscles of the feet also contributes to poor venous return, since walking, which is another mechanism to assist in venous return to the heart, is curtailed. Absence of these mechanisms allows a rise to occur in the intraluminal leg vein pressure. Higher venous pressure in the ankle and foot allows more fluid to pass into the tissues and overloads the lymphatic system so they are unable to function as required.[22]

Neuropathic Ulcer Grading

The Wagner dysvascular foot classification system is the most widely used system for grading neuropathic ulcers (Table 2-2). Recently, its readability, validity, and reliability have been evaluated.[23] A systematic review comparing the Wagner system with other newer classification systems concluded that there are deficits and complicating factors in each of the systems. Although there is scant evidence of validity of the Wagner system, it may be appropriate to use as a guide for treatment and prognosis of patients with ulcers as a result of neuropathy, but knowing that the classification has less reliability for other patient populations. One of the most significant faults of the Wagner scale is the absence of indicators, such as biomechanics, foot deformity, ulcer size, infection, and presence of peripheral vascular disease.[23] All of these factors have been shown to impact ulcer development, healing, and risk of amputation.[21] Other deficits include the omission of circulatory and neuropathy factors. Grade 0 is used to evaluate for predisposing factors leading to breakdown, and Grades 1 through 3 are used for risk management. Treatment usually is geared toward pressure relief and/or circulatory management for Grades 0 to 1 that are diabetic pre-ulcerative conditions.[21,24]

The University of Texas-San Antonio classification system (Table 2-3) is being used in situations where more information is desired about infection, circulation (PVD), and the combination of infection and ischemia in order to assign risk and predict outcomes in patients with neuropathic ulcerations.[25] However, it also lacks consideration of the biomechanics and neuropathy. Analysis of the system found that it is a better predictor of group outcome than of individual patient outcome.

Spinal Cord Injury

The individual with a spinal cord lesion has loss of sensation below the level of injury and may be unable to reposition, which may put this individual at risk for pressure ulcers. Autonomic dysreflexia often encountered in individuals with spinal cord injury (SCI) below T6 may also contribute to decreased blood flow in the peripheral microcirculation, thus potentially increasing susceptibility to pressure sores.[26] Pooling of blood in the paralyzed LEs contributes to venous insufficiency and edema. These common complications put the integument of the legs at risk for breakdown.

Shear forces contribute to mechanical destruction of tissue usually from the deep soft tissue-bone interface, which is often observed as superficial skin disruption before breaking down into a deep pressure ulcer. Friction occurs when the skin and another surface rub across each other. This traumatizes the protective outer layers of the skin. Individuals with SCI who have difficulty with repositioning or who are pulled across the bed linen may experience this wearing away of the outer layer of the skin. Friction and shear act together to increase risk of pressure ulcers over the sacro-coccygeal area.[27]

Immunosuppression

Individuals who have compromised immune systems include those who are HIV positive, have diabetes with high glucose levels, have cancer, are receiving chemotherapy and/or radiation, and are on anti-inflammatory and steroidal drugs. All of these factors are known to impede wound healing either by inhibiting the initial inflammatory response or by disruption of the normal healing progression.[28]

Chronic Obstructive Pulmonary Disease

Patients with COPD are often on medications, such as steroids, that impair the body's ability to mount an adequate inflammatory response. This ultimately affects one's ability to initiate the healing cascade and to keep it functioning adequately for tissue repair to occur.

Nutritional Status

Adequate nutrition includes sufficient calories, proteins, fluids, vitamins, and minerals to maintain good health. Caloric needs are usually met with 30 to 35 kilocalories per kilogram of body weight per day. Recommended protein intake to meet metabolic needs is 1.25 to 1.5 grams of protein per kilogram of body weight per day. Minimal fluid needs are 1500 mL daily, which is generally met by taking 30 mL/kg of body weight per day or an amount equal to kilocalorie requirements.[29] The terminology "poor nutritional status" is preferred to "malnutrition," because it is a more descriptive and inclusive term. Some signs of poor nutritional status include[30]:

- ♦ Hair: Dull, dry, sparse, easily plucked
- ♦ Eyes: Redness or fissures at the eyelid corners
- ♦ Lips: Redness and swelling
- ♦ Face: Pallor, scaling of skin around nostrils
- ♦ Mental status: Confusion
- ♦ Unintended weight loss
  - 10% in 6 months
  - 7.5% in 3 months
  - 5% in 30 days
  - More than 2% in 7 days

Nutrition markers linked to skin breakdown and wound healing include serum albumin and prealbumin, and both are regarded as diagnostic of nutritional status.

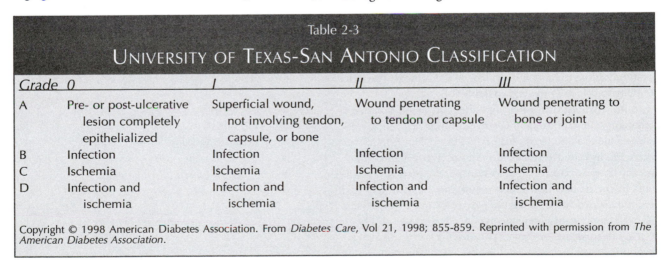

	Grade 0	I	II	III
A	Pre- or post-ulcerative lesion completely epithelialized	Superficial wound, not involving tendon, capsule, or bone	Wound penetrating to tendon or capsule	Wound penetrating to bone or joint
B	Infection	Infection	Infection	Infection
C	Ischemia	Ischemia	Ischemia	Ischemia
D	Infection and ischemia	Infection and ischemia	Infection and ischemia	Infection and ischemia

Table 2-3

UNIVERSITY OF TEXAS-SAN ANTONIO CLASSIFICATION

Copyright © 1998 American Diabetes Association. From *Diabetes Care*, Vol 21, 1998; 855-859. Reprinted with permission from *The American Diabetes Association*.

Table 2-4	
SERUM ALBUMIN LEVELS	
>3.5 g/dL	Normal level
3.0 to 3.5 g/dL	Mild depletion
2.5 to 3.0 g/dL	Moderate depletion
<2.5 g/dL	Severe depletion

Table 2-5	
PREALBUMIN LEVELS	
15 to 43 mg/dL	Normal nutrition
11 to 14.9 mg/dL	Increased risk
5 to 10.9 mg/dL	Significant nutritional risk
0 to 5 mg/dL	Severe depletion

Serum albumin has a half-life of about 12 to 18 days. Concentration of serum albumin falls slowly with malnutrition, but it increases with dehydration. Serum albumin levels decrease when there is overhydration, liver disease, malnutrition, infection, stress, pressure ulcers, severe burns, surgery, cytokine-induced inflammatory states, patients older than 70 years of age, and the like.[30] Deficit levels of serum albumin can be classified as shown in Table 2-4.[31]

Prealbumin is a measure of protein in the blood with a half-life of 2 to 3 days and is used as an early indicator of poor nutritional status.[30-32] Elevated prealbumin levels may indicate renal failure, dehydration, Hodgkin's lymphoma, or pregnancy. Decreased levels may indicate liver disease, malnutrition, catabolic states, metabolic stress, inflammation, surgical trauma, hyperthyroidism, and cytokine-induced inflammatory states. Table 2-5 provides the range of prealbumin levels.[30-32]

Hydration

Water is an essential nutrient for life. Maintaining water levels or hydration is accomplished by daily replacement of fluids. Fluid requirements are usually met with 30 mL/kg of body weight or a minimum of 1500 mL per day unless there are adverse health issues, such as fever, diarrhea, vomiting, or sweating. When these conditions exist, the daily requirements for water increase.[29] Water serves multiple functions including providing blood volume to transport oxygen and nutrients to the tissue to prevent infection and heal tissues.[28] It acts as a solvent for minerals, vitamins, amino acids, glucose, and other important elements enabling them to diffuse in and out of the cells. Waste products are transported away with water. Water also serves as a lubricant of the joints and as a means of controlling body temperature.[33] When fluid intake does not match fluid output, the result may be dehydration leading to fluid and electrolyte imbalances. The signs of dehydration are provided in Table 2-6.[33]

Since hydration is a key ingredient in blood volume, a laboratory measure to quantify hydration is helpful. A measure of blood volume or volemia is Hct. A Hct level of less than 33% is below normal and indicates hypovolemia, which means there is limited fluid to transport oxygen and nutrients to the tissues. Low blood volume may potentially lead to an increased risk of integumentary damage. Hypovolemia is more significant than anemia in altering the ability to transport adequate oxygen and nutrients to the tissues for healing.[28]

Obesity

Obesity may be associated with protein malnutrition. Adipose tissue has a poor blood supply, and an adequate blood supply is important for healing. In addition, obesity has been identified as a risk factor for integumentary breakdown due to pressure on the venous system with progression to changes in the integument of the LEs as described under venous insufficiency.[34]

Allergies

Tapes, antibiotic ointments, and latex are some common sources of allergic reactions that may result in urticaria or erythema. One must rule out allergic reactions as a source of superficial skin irritation.

EXTRINSIC FACTORS ASSOCIATED WITH RISK OF INTEGUMENTARY IMPAIRMENTS

Medications including steroids, immunosuppressive agents, antineoplastic agents, and anticoagulants (including aspirin and NSAIDs) are associated with poor integumentary recovery from injury.[28] Pattern A: Primary Prevention/Risk Reduction for Integumentary Disorders details these medications.

Irradiation produces changes in skin, specifically in the treatment field, immediately or subsequently, and has life-long risks. Clinical manifestations include skin irritations, dryness with possible peeling, itching, swelling, thinning, rashes, and possibly moist, weepy areas. Following radiation long-term skin care is needed. Skin care should include daily

Table 2-6
SIGNS OF DEHYDRATION
♦ Dry mouth
♦ Dry, cracked lips
♦ Sunken eyes
♦ Dark urine
♦ Poor skin turgor
♦ Increased confusion
♦ Increased blood glucose levels

Adapted from Posthaur ME. Nutritional assessment and treatment. In: Sussman C, Bates-Jensen BM, ed. *Would Care: A Collaborative Practice Manual for Physical Therapists and Nurses.* 2nd ed. Gaithersburg, Md: Aspen Publishers, Inc; 2001:52-76.

moisturizing, use of sunscreen (SPF 15 or greater), and protection from irritants. Irritants include cleaning solutions, solvents, friction and shear from clothing, scratching, and extremes of heat and cold.[35]

Psychophysiologic stress has been identified as playing a significant role in impaired wound healing and in skin breakdown.[36,37] Stress accounts for activation of the sympathetic nervous system and subsequent release of adrenalin, noradrenalin, and cortisol. Increased cortisol levels block migration of neutrophils and inhibit the synthesis of proinflammatory mediators creating interference during the early inflammatory stage.[10] Stress also depletes nutritional stores, which compromises integumentary recovery from a wound.[38]

Incontinence, a loss of bladder or bowel control, releases chemical irritants onto the skin that can lead to maceration and is a source of bacterial contamination and fungal problems.[27] Incontinence or peritoneal dermatitis is sometimes misdiagnosed as a Stage I pressure ulcer. There are a number of factors that may contribute to urinary incontinence.[39] Altered mental status may be a signal of urinary tract infection often accompanied by increased urgency. Pharmaceuticals affect continence either by reducing the person's ability to recognize and respond appropriately to bladder filling or altering the contractility of the bladder. Many individuals are on diuretic medications that may cause a sense of urgency leading to urinary incontinence. Restricted mobility or dexterity that reduces the ability to use the toilet is another contributing factor to incontinence. Mixed fecal and urinary incontinence occur frequently together, and in those cases management of fecal incontinence is the priority. Incontinence has been identified as an important risk factor in the development of pressure ulcers.[27] Identification and treatment of reversible causes of incontinence are the recommended strategies. Physical therapist strategies for treatment of incontinence are found in Musculoskeletal Pattern B, Case Study #2. Therapeutic skin care for incontinence dermatitis includes use of a gentle cleanser, treatment of reddened irritated skin with therapeutic cream or ointments, and protection of the skin against continued irritation with a moisture barrier.

The pathogenesis of bacterial burden or infection of the superficial skin includes viruses, bacteria, fungi, or parasites.[40] In general, the clinical manifestations of most skin infections include erythema, edema, focal accumulations of pus- or fluid-filled vesicles or bullae, scaling with no apparent inflammation, discoloration of nails, and thickening of the nail plate. These manifestations may vary from disease to disease. Microbiologic examination is used to make the differential diagnosis. The resistance of the host, the virulence of the organism toxin, and the number of bacteria determine whether infection will occur. Of these factors, the host resistance is the most important factor.[41]

Pressure, including friction and shear, significantly affects superficial integumentary integrity. Pressure ulcer definition includes areas of local tissue trauma that usually develop where soft tissues are compressed between a bony prominence and any external surface for a long period of time resulting in irreversible ischemia.[42] Constant pressure for over 2 hours can produce a pressure ulcer. A shearing force affects mainly the deep tissues at the attachment of the bone to the soft tissues. Shearing forces occur when the body skeleton "slides into the skin" (eg, a patient sliding down in a chair or in a bed if head is elevated above 30 degrees).[43,44] Friction is created by two surfaces moving across one another (eg, pulling a patient across bed linen). Friction and shear are exacerbated in individuals with spastic conditions or those who have difficulty sitting up without sliding down while in a bedside chair or wheelchair. Friction and shear together contribute to pressure ulcers especially in the area of the coccyx.

There appears to be an inverse relationship between the amount of pressure exerted and amount of time before tissue is damaged.[27] Clinical appearance of a pressure ulcer in intact skin (National Pressure Ulcer Advisory Panel [NPUAP] Stage I)[45] is characterized by unblanchable erythema in lightly pigmented skin or darkening of skin in persons of color. This is often the first manifestation of tissue damage. Pain and temperature changes may also be present. Violescent color of intact skin may indicate deep tissue trauma that has not yet manifested as deep ulceration. The area of trauma may be identified by a well-defined border between the area of color change and the surrounding skin. Pressure ulcers, which are staged, are consider to be preventable in most cases.[46] A pressure ulcer staging system has been adopted by the Agency of Healthcare Policy and Research Pressure Ulcer Guideline Panels and is published in both sets of AHCPR (now known as the Agency for Healthcare Quality and Research) Pressure Ulcer Clinical Practice Guidelines.[42,43] The Stage I definition was revised in 1997.[45] Table 2-7 delineates the NPUAP Pressure Ulcer Staging System.[45,46]

LIFESTYLE AND INAPPROPRIATE WOUND CARE

Smoking contributes to vasoconstriction and ischemic conditions of the integument and underlying tissues and is also related to increased metalloproteases.[47] Exercise has positive benefits on the prevention of integumentary breakdown. For example, exercise complements compression therapy in the presence of venous disease, because the muscle pumping action improves circulation to affected tissues. However, care must be taken during exercise to avoid stress on painful tissues.

Dressing products have both positive and negative attributes. Adhesives may strip the stratum corneum from the skin making the skin permeable to external substances.[1] Dressing products should be checked so as not to maintain excessive moisture on the skin surface and cause maceration.

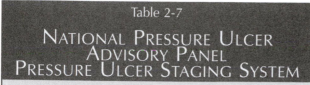

Table 2-7

NATIONAL PRESSURE ULCER ADVISORY PANEL PRESSURE ULCER STAGING SYSTEM

Stage I: Pressure ulcer is an observable pressure-related alteration of intact skin whose indicators as compared to an adjacent or opposite area on the body may include changes in one or more of the following: skin temperature (warmth or coolness), tissue consistency (firm or boggy feel), and/or sensation (pain, itching). The ulcer appears as a defined area of persistent redness in lightly pigmented skin, whereas in darker skin tones, the ulcer may appear with persistent red, blue, or purple hues.*

Stage II: Partial-thickness skin loss involving epidermis, dermis, or both. The ulcer is superficial and presents clinically as an abrasion, blister, or shallow crater.**

Stage III: Full-thickness skin loss involving damage to, or necrosis of, subcutaneous tissue that may extend down to, but not through, underlying fascia. The ulcer presents clinically as a deep crater with or without undermining of adjacent tissue.**

Stage IV: Full-thickness skin loss with extensive destruction, tissue necrosis, or damage to muscle, bone, or supporting structures (eg, tendon, joint, capsule). Undermining and sinus tracts also may be associated with Stage IV pressure ulcers.**

*Adapted from Henderson C, Ayello C, Sussman C. Draft definition of stage I pressure ulcers: inclusion of person with darkly pigmented skin. *Advances in Skin and Wound Care*. 1997;10:34-35.
**Adapted from National Pressure Ulcer Advisory Panel. Pressure ulcers, prevalence, cost, and risk assessment: consensus development conference statement. *Decubitus*. 1989;2(2):24-28.

It is important to select dressing products that maintain the moisture balance of the impaired skin—not too dry or overhydrated.[48]

PHARMACOLOGY

- Skin sealants and moisture barriers
  - Examples: Skin-Prep, SensiCare, 3M No Sting Skin Protectant
  - Actions: Form a protective layer or coating over the skin to prevent water, body fluids, or antimicrobial topical agents from irritating periwound tissue or as prevention to urine and fecal incontinence
  - Administered: Topically to the at-risk tissue
  - Side effects: Skin irritation

CONCLUSION

The skin functions as a barrier to protect the body from the external environment. Intact skin keeps moisture and nutrients in and debris and undesirable organisms out. The health of the skin provides a window to the internal health of the host and the ability to withstand skin breakdown. Conversely, the health of the host is a predictor of potential for skin breakdown. Protection of the health and well-being of intact skin is essential for good health.

Case Study #1: First-Degree Burn written by Betsy A. Myers, PT, MPT, MHS, OCS, CLT

Justin Wiley is a 16-year-old male who has burns due to a splash injury (Figure 2-1).

PHYSICAL THERAPIST EXAMINATION

HISTORY

- General demographics: Justin Wiley is a 16-year-old male whose primary language is English. He is right-hand dominant and is a high school junior.
- Social history: Justin lives with his stepmother and father.
- Employment/work: Justin is a full-time student and works 10 hours a week as a dishwasher in a local restaurant.
- Living environment: Justin shares a room with his younger brother in a two-story house with three steps to enter.
- General health status
  - General health perception: He reports that his health status is good.
  - Physical function: He reports no physical limitations.
  - Role function: Student, musician, athlete.
  - Social function: Justin plays the guitar in the high school jazz band and is on the swim team. He has a 16-year-old girlfriend who is also on the swim team.
- Social/health habits: Justin is a nondrinker and non-smoker. He exercises 3 days a week in physical education class and has swim practice twice daily 5 days a week during the current preseason.
- Family history: Justin reports his mother died after complications from a house fire when he was 4 years

old. His father has high BP. His grandparents are all living. His paternal grandfather has been diagnosed with Alzheimer's disease.

♦ Medical/surgical history: His history is unremarkable. He has had all childhood vaccines and has had a recent tetanus shot. Justin had the chicken pox at age 8.

♦ Current condition(s)/chief complaint(s): Justin complains of a painful burn from a splash injury that occurred about 2 hours ago. His father is concerned the burn may be serious. Justin is concerned he will be unable to swim in the preseason swim meet next week and that the wound will cause extensive scarring. No wound treatment has been rendered at this time.

♦ Functional status and activity level: Justin reports no limitations in IADL, although he is unsure how he will be able to swim with a burn.

♦ Medications: Justin was given a prescription by the emergency room physician for a 3-day supply of hydrocodone for pain if needed.

SYSTEMS REVIEW

♦ Cardiovascular/pulmonary
  • BP: 135/89 mmHg
  • Edema: None
  • HR: 84 bpm
  • RR: 10 bpm
♦ Integumentary
  • Presence of scar formation: None
  • Skin color: Wounds with erythema, all else unremarkable
  • Skin integrity: Burn anterior R thorax and R forearm
♦ Musculoskeletal
  • Gross range of motion: WNL
  • Gross strength: BLE/UE grossly 5/5
  • Gross symmetry: Symmetrical
  • Height: 6'1" (1.85 m)
  • Weight: 144 lbs (4.08 kg)
♦ Neuromuscular
  • Transfers independently
  • Gait independent
♦ Communication, affect, cognition, language, and learning style
  • Communication, affect, cognition: WNL
  • Learning preferences: Patient and father learn best by reviewing written information

TESTS AND MEASURES

♦ Anthropometric characteristics
  • BMI=19, which is normal
♦ Assistive and adaptive devices: None used

Figure 2-1. Superficial splash wound. Reprinted with permission from Myers B. *Wound Management: Principles and Practice.* Atlanta, Ga: Pearson Education; 2003. (See this figure in the Color Atlas following page 39.)

♦ Circulation
  • Pulse exam[49-51] (see Tables 2-3 and 3-4)
    ▪ Performed as an indicator of arterial blood flow
    ▪ UEs and LEs=2+
  • Capillary refill[52-58] (see Table 3-5)
    ▪ Performed as an indicator of superficial blood flow
    ▪ 2 seconds bilaterally
♦ Cranial and peripheral nerve integrity (see Table 4-5)
  • Semmes-Weinstein monofilament testing
    ▪ Performed to assess sensation and as an alternative indicator of depth of burn injury
    ▪ He is able to detect 5.07 monofilament on his anterior thorax and both forearms
♦ Gait, locomotion, and balance
  • He is independent in transfers
  • During ambulation, he tends to slightly flex his trunk
♦ Integumentary integrity
  • Associated skin
    ▪ Skin color: Erythema in wound areas
    ▪ Hair growth: Normal
    ▪ Nail growth: Normal
    ▪ Temperature: Burns are slightly warm to palpation
    ▪ Texture/turgor: Normal
    ▪ Edema: None
  • Wound (see Figure 2-1)
    ▪ Irregular-shaped wounds on right anterior thorax and right forearm
    ▪ Skin barrier function is intact
    ▪ Burn covers approximately 5.5% total body surface area[62]
    ▪ Burn drainage: None

♦ Muscle performance
  • Unimpaired when assessed by way of manual muscle testing
  • Justin notes testing of right wrist flexors increases his forearm pain
♦ Pain
  • Justin rates his wound pain as a 4/10 on the VAS[59-61]
♦ Range of motion: Unimpaired
♦ Work, community, and leisure integration or reintegration
  • Justin reports concern about his ability to swim in the preseason swim meet in 9 days and is concerned about scarring
  • Justin's father reports concern about infection and Justin's ability to return to school

EVALUATION

Justin's history and risk factors previously outlined indicate that he is a healthy, physically active young male who sustained a splash burn covering approximately 5.5% of his body located over his right thorax and right forearm. He has limitations in swimming and self-care.

DIAGNOSIS

Justin has sustained a superficial splash burn over his right thorax and right forearm. He has impaired circulation and integumentary integrity. He is functionally limited in work, community, and leisure actions, tasks, and activities. His ability to return to school in the morning is unknown. These findings are consistent with placement in Pattern B: Impaired Integumentary Integrity Associated With Superficial Skin Involvement.[63] These impairments and functional limitations will be addressed in determining the prognosis and the plan of care.

PROGNOSIS AND PLAN OF CARE

Over the course of one to six visits, the following mutually established outcomes have been determined:
♦ Ability to perform leisure activities is improved
♦ Ability to perform self-care and return to work activities (school) are improved
♦ Patient/family knowledge and awareness of diagnosis, prognosis, interventions, and anticipated goals and outcomes are increased
♦ Risk of secondary impairment is reduced
♦ Skin integrity is restored

To achieve these outcomes, the appropriate interventions for this patient are determined. These will include: coordi-

nation, communication, and documentation; patient/client-related instruction; functional training in self-care and home management; functional training in work, community, and leisure integration or reintegration; and integumentary repair and protection techniques.

Based on the diagnosis and prognosis, Justin is expected to require between five to six visits over a 2-week period of time. Justin is young, is motivated, and follows through with his home program. He is not severely impaired and is healthy.

INTERVENTIONS

RATIONALE FOR SELECTED INTERVENTIONS

Integumentary Repair and Protection Techniques

Integumentary repair and protection techniques for Justin will include the use of a moisturizer to decrease pruritis and improve skin pliability. Physical agents, such as whirlpool or pulsatile lavage, are not indicated as the skin barrier function is intact and no slough, eschar, or foreign debris is present. Wound dressings are not required as the skin barrier function is intact.

COORDINATION, COMMUNICATION, AND DOCUMENTATION

Care will be coordinated with Justin's father. All elements of the patient's management will be documented.

PATIENT/CLIENT-RELATED INSTRUCTION

Justin and his father will be instructed in normal burn wound healing. Particular emphasis will be placed on:
♦ Superficial burns have an intact skin barrier function. Therefore, the risk of infection is no greater than prior to the burn injury
♦ Superficial burns resolve without scarring spontaneously within 3 to 5 days[64,65]
♦ Skin exfoliation may occur[66] within the first 2 to 5 days after a superficial burn
♦ Pain can be expected to decrease rapidly over the next 24 to 48 hours
♦ Proper burn management
♦ Avoiding skin trauma by:
  • Protecting against friction, as may occur from pant waistband
  • Not scratching the burned areas
  • Limiting sun exposure to burn wounds until erythema resolves.

Because Justin and his father learn best by reading, patient education will be reinforced with written instructions.

FUNCTIONAL TRAINING IN SELF-CARE AND HOME MANAGEMENT

- ◆ Home management
  - Wear loose fitting, nonabrasive clothing until burn wounds heal
  - Bathe wound daily

FUNCTIONAL TRAINING IN WORK, COMMUNITY, AND LEISURE INTEGRATION OR REINTEGRATION

- ◆ Work (school)
  - Return to regular school schedule the day after the physical therapy examination
- ◆ Leisure
  - Do not participate in pool portions of swim practice until no longer taking hydrocodone
  - Temporary alternative methods of training, if needed, may include:
    - Weight training
    - Aerobic exercise
      - ▸ Upper body ergometry
      - ▸ Bicycle
      - ▸ Treadmill
      - ▸ Stair climber
    - If swimming in an outdoor pool or exposing erythematous skin to strong sunlight, apply sunscreen to affected areas to protect the skin from further trauma
    - Apply moisturizing agent after showering upon completion of swim practice

INTEGUMENTARY REPAIR AND PROTECTION TECHNIQUES

- ◆ Topical agents
  - The burns should be gently cleansed with soap and water during regular daily bathing and patted dry
  - An over-the-counter moisturizer may be applied gently two or more times per day over the burn wounds on the anterior thorax and right forearm to decrease pruritis and improve skin pliability

ANTICIPATED GOALS AND EXPECTED OUTCOMES

- ◆ Impact on pathology/pathophysiology
  - Pain is decreased to 0/10 after 1 week.
- ◆ Impact on impairments
  - Integumentary integrity is improved, burn is healed in 1 week.
- ◆ Impact on functional limitations
  - Performance levels in self-care, home management, work, community, or leisure actions, tasks, and activities are improved, and independence is achieved in all activities in 1 week.
  - Tolerance to positions or activities is increased and is unlimited by burn in 1 week.
- ◆ Risk reduction/prevention
  - Self-management of symptoms is improved and includes independence with moisturizer application in one visit.
- ◆ Impact on health, wellness, and fitness
  - Physical function is improved.
- ◆ Impact on societal resources
  - Documentation occurs throughout patient management and follows APTA's *Guidelines for Physical Therapy Documentation.*[63]
  - Care is coordinated with patient/family and other professionals.
- ◆ Patient/client satisfaction
  - Patient and family understanding of anticipated goals and expected outcomes is increased.
  - Patient/family knowledge and awareness of the diagnosis, prognosis, interventions, and anticipated goals and expected outcomes are increased.

REEXAMINATION

Reexamination is performed throughout the episode of care.

DISCHARGE

Justin Wiley is discharged from physical therapy after a total of four sessions and attainment of his goals and expectations. These sessions have covered his entire episode of care. He is discharged because he has achieved his goals and expected outcomes.

PSYCHOLOGICAL ASPECTS

Given the Wileys' previous experience with burn wounds, it is extremely important to reassure Justin and his father that the normal course of superficial burn healing is complete resolution of symptoms within 3 to 5 days without further skilled interventions. Because Justin is a young swimmer, he may be concerned that the burn will heal with scar formation and that it will be noticed by his girlfriend, teammates, or competitors. He should be reassured that superficial burns heal without scar formation and that the erythema will resolve quickly. If he is concerned about exposing his burn to his teammates and girlfriend, he may want to wear a t-shirt during swim practice until the symptoms resolve.

Case Study #2:
Stage I Pressure Ulcer

Jim Clark is an 80-year-old male, long-term care resident, with a diagnosis of cerebral vascular accident with right hemiparesis and with a painful reddened area on the right buttock.

PHYSICAL THERAPIST EXAMINATION

HISTORY

♦ General demographics: Mr. Clark is an 80-year-old white male who had a high school education. His primary language is English.

♦ Social history: Mr. Clark is widowed and has two sons who live nearby but are not involved with his care. His granddaughter visits regularly.

♦ Employment/work: Mr. Clark worked as a longshoreman for many years and has been retired for 15 years.

♦ General health status
  ● General health perception: Mr. Clark reports that his health status is poor.
  ● Physical function: His physical function is impaired requiring assistance for ADL.
  ● Psychological function: Mr. Clark is alert but unable to express himself clearly due to expressive aphasia. He appears to be depressed.
  ● Role function: Father, grandfather, long-term care resident for 2 years.
  ● Social function: He liked being with his friends in the long-term care facility and used to play cards but has lost that interest and ability since his cerebral vascular accident (CVA).

♦ Social/health habits: Mr. Clark was a smoker for 40 years at one to two packs/day. He stopped 5 years ago.

♦ Family history: His mother had a stroke when she was age 65 and died 2 years later. His father died at age 59 from colon cancer.

♦ Medical/surgical history: He experienced a CVA with right upper extremity (RUE) hemiplegia and RLE hemiparesis 3 weeks prior to this evaluation.

♦ Prior hospitalizations: Mr. Clark had colon polyps removed 10 years ago. He had a right hip fracture with hip internal fixation 2 years ago after which he had difficulty walking and taking care of himself. That is when he entered the long-term care facility.

♦ Preexisting medical and other health-related conditions: He has a chronic cough. Mr. Clark also has a history of falls.

♦ Current condition(s)/chief complaint(s): Mr. Clark finds sitting in his wheelchair produces pain in his buttocks. He is unable to stand up to relieve the discomfort and shifting position in the wheelchair makes it worse.

♦ Functional status and activity level: He is moderately dependent in all ADL and IADL.

♦ Medications: Mr. Clark is taking 1000 mg of calcium/day, multivitamins, and blood thinner (Coumadin).

♦ Other clinical tests: His albumin and prealbumin levels are both in the low range as was his Hgb and Hct (see Table 3-10).
  ● Albumin=3.4 mg/dL
  ● Prealbumin=13 mg/dL
  ● Hgb=11.8 g/dL
  ● Hct=33%

SYSTEMS REVIEW

♦ Cardiovascular/pulmonary
  ● BP: 140/82 mmHg
  ● Edema: None
  ● HR: 64 bpm
  ● RR: 16 bpm

♦ Integumentary
  ● Presence of scar formation: Scar from surgery to R hip following fracture and internal fixation 2 years ago is healed
  ● Skin color: WNL except for nonblanchable erythema on right buttock over ischial tuberosity which corresponds to the NPUAP definition of a Stage I pressure ulcer in white skin
  ● Skin integrity: Intact

♦ Musculoskeletal
  ● Gross range of motion
    ■ RUE moderately limited
    ■ RLE mildly limited
  ● Gross strength
    ■ Moderately limited RUE (fair to poor)
    ■ Minimally limited RLE (fair to good)
  ● Gross symmetry: Asymmetrical
  ● Height: 5'8" (1.73 m)
  ● Weight: 140 lbs (63.5 kg)

♦ Neuromuscular
  ● Balance: Moderately unsteady
  ● Locomotion, transfers, and transitions: With moderate assist, transitions subject to friction and shear

♦ Communication, affect, cognition, language, and learning style
  ● Communication, affect, and cognition limited due

to expressive aphasia, flat affect, mildly impaired cognition

- Learning preferences: Auditory learner

TESTS AND MEASURES

- ◆ Anthropometric characteristics
  - BMI: Weight 140 lb x 700 divided by height[2] (5'8"=68") BMI=18.16 which is considered underweight (range of normal=18.5 to 24.9)
- ◆ Arousal, attention, and cognition
  - OEE indicated awareness of exercise benefits
- ◆ Cranial and peripheral nerve integrity
  - Ability to detect pain and both light and deep pressure over bony prominences revealed:
    - Diminished sensation that increases risk of skin breakdown
  - Pressure
    - Pressure sensation is intact on L side of body
    - Diminished pressure sensation over the R buttock and LE
- ◆ Ergonomics and body mechanics
  - Analysis of body mechanics during bed positioning, transfers, and while up in wheelchair revealed:
    - Difficulty sitting erect and slumping
    - Asymmetry with right side leaning
    - Scoots buttocks forward in chair frequently
  - Poor postural awareness
- ◆ Gait, locomotion, and balance
  - Sit to stand requires moderate assist
  - Balance is fair in stance
  - During gait with walker, R foot lags and needs support device for RUE
- ◆ Integumentary integrity
  - Risk assessment
    - Mr. Clark's total score is 16/23 on the Braden scale
    - Braden has ranked protocols for prevention by risk score[67]
    - A total score of 16 puts Mr. Clark at a mild risk for pressure ulcer
    - Therefore, a Stage I pressure/friction ulcer on his seating surface should have been preventable[42]
  - Computerized pressure mapping device shows high areas of pressure over the ischial tuberosities R>L while seated in wheelchair
- ◆ Motor function
  - Observation of dexterity, coordination, and agility revealed activities are impaired on the right side of body
- ◆ Muscle performance
  - Dynamometry revealed grip strength of 10 kg (nor-

mal 23 kg) of dominant right side

- Manual muscle tests revealed the following deviations from normal
  - Thoracic spine extension=3/5
  - Lower abdominals=2/5
  - Scapular adduction R=3/5, L=3/5
  - Scapula depression R=3/5, L=3/5
  - UE shoulder flexion R=2+/5, L=4/5
  - UE shoulder extension R=2/5, L=4/5
  - UE shoulder abduction R=2/5, L=4/5
  - UE shoulder external rotation R=2/5, L=4/5
  - LE hip abduction R=3-/5, L=4/5
  - LE hip extension R=3-/5, L=4+/5
- ◆ Pain
  - Pain severity reported as 4/6 using the Faces Pain scale (0=no pain and 6=worst pain or agony)
    - The patient chooses the face on the scale that best describes how he feels
    - The Faces Pain scale may be more appropriate for use with the elderly, children, and those with cognitive deficits or who do not speak or understand English[68]
  - Pain in R buttock continuous but more severe with sitting >30 minutes
- ◆ Posture
  - Observational assessment and grid photographs revealed
    - Forward head
    - Moderately increased thoracic spine lateral bend toward R
    - Moderately decreased lumbar spine lordosis
    - Moderate pronation R foot
    - Pes planus
- ◆ Self-care and home management
  - Requires moderate assist for self-care
- ◆ Work, community, and leisure integration or reintegration
  - Interview concerning ability to manage leisure activities and tasks revealed that they could be done, but difficulty as noted with depression, communication, and dexterity of RUE

EVALUATION

Mr. Clark's history and risk factors previously outlined indicated that he is an elderly male, previous smoker, nonexerciser, and has been living in a long-term care facility since his hip fracture surgery 2 years ago. His BMI of 18.16 signifies low/borderline poor nutritional status. He has nonblanchable erythema and pain over his R ischial tuberosity consistent with the classification of a Stage I pressure ulcer probably caused by friction and shear in the wheelchair and during transfers. He has asymmetrical right leaning sitting posture, impaired standing balance, impaired standing posture with right side leaning, and impaired motor performance in his RUE, both LEs, and trunk. He also has difficulty with ADL and IADL.

DIAGNOSIS

Mr. Clark is a patient with superficial skin involvement with pain over the R ischial tuberosity (a Stage I pressure ulcer over the R ischial tuberosity). He has a Braden scale that indicates mild risk[42,67] for pressure ulcer formation, a low BMI, and albumin and prealbumin levels that are indicators of poor nutritional status. He has impaired: anthropometric characteristics; cranial and peripheral nerve integrity; ergonomics and body mechanics; gait, locomotion, and balance; integumentary integrity; motor function; motor performance; and posture. He is functionally limited in self-care and home management and in work, community, and leisure actions, tasks, and activities. He is in need of adaptive and assistive devices and equipment. These findings are consistent with placement in Pattern B: Impaired Integumentary Integrity Associated With Superficial Skin Involvement.[63] He will also be classified in Neuromuscular Pattern D: Impaired Motor Function and Sensory Integrity Associated With Nonprogressive Disorders of the Central Nervous System—Acquired in Adolescence or Adulthood.[63] These impairments, functional limitations, and adaptive and assistive device needs will be addressed in determining the prognosis and the plan of care.

PROGNOSIS AND PLAN OF CARE

Over the course of the visits, the following mutually established outcomes have been determined:
♦ Adaptive devices, including an appropriate pressure relief mattress and wheelchair cushion, will reduce risk of skin breakdown
♦ Knowledge of behaviors that foster healthy habits, wellness, and prevention is increased
♦ Pain in buttock is reduced
♦ Postural control and spinal proprioception are improved
♦ Pressure ulcer nonblanchable erythema is resolved
♦ Right buttock area blood flow is increased
♦ Risk of secondary impairment (such as new pressure ulcers and increased pressure ulcer severity) is reduced
♦ Sitting posture symmetry is improved
♦ Transfer techniques are improved, and shear and friction are minimized
To achieve these outcomes, the appropriate interventions for this patient are determined. These will include: coordi-

nation, communication, and documentation; patient/client-related instruction; therapeutic exercise; functional training in self-care and home management; functional training in work, community, and leisure integration or reintegration; prescription, application, and, as appropriate, fabrication of devices and equipment; integumentary repair and protection techniques; and electrotherapeutic modalities.

Based on the diagnosis and prognosis, Mr. Clark is expected to require four to six visits over a 3-week period of time. Mr. Clark is a resident of a long-term care facility who will need to follow up on his care needs.

INTERVENTIONS

RATIONALE FOR SELECTED INTERVENTIONS

Therapeutic Exercise

Exercise is an intervention that may also address other impairments associated with his condition of limited mobility. His stroke is only 3 weeks post onset, and he would be a candidate for a rehabilitation program for this health problem. See Neuromuscular Pattern D: Impaired Motor Function and Sensory Integrity Associated With Nonprogressive Disorders of the Central Nervous System—Acquired in Adolescence or Adulthood.[63]

Prescription, Application, and, as Appropriate, Fabrication of Devices and Equipment

Rationale for use of positioning devices and pressure reduction devices may be found in Pattern A: Primary Prevention/Risk Reduction for Integumentary Disorders, Case Study #1.

Integumentary Repair and Protection Techniques

Patients at risk for pressure ulcer development or with an identified Stage I pressure ulcer may benefit from the use of sealants if incontinence or moisture is a concern.[35,43,64]

Electrotherapeutic Modalities

Transcutaneous electrical nerve stimulation (TENS) will increase blood flow and promote absorption of edema and bring oxygen and nutrients to the tissues. The efficacy of the use of TENS for increasing blood flow is supported in multiple research studies,[69-72] as is the efficacy of TENS to modulate pain.[73,74]

COORDINATION, COMMUNICATION, AND DOCUMENTATION

Communication will occur with Mr. Clark, his family members, and other members of the long-term care team to engender support for his therapeutic positioning and mobility program. A referral to a nutritionist/dietitian will be made to ensure appropriate diet for enhancing tissue repair and prevention of skin breakdown. Referral back to the physician will be made for management of his depression problem. A speech and language pathologist referral would be made for the aphasia communication problem and possible dysphagia. The occupational therapist will be made aware that the deficits in self-care increase his risk for skin breakdown. All elements of the patient's management will be documented.

PATIENT/CLIENT-RELATED INSTRUCTION

The patient will be instructed in the risk factors related to pressure ulcers, the importance of pressure relief, and the need to eat an adequate diet. Mr. Clark's caregivers will understand the importance of therapeutic positioning in bed and in his wheelchair with respect to the prevention of skin breakdown and further development of pressure ulcers. Stress as a result of illness (eg, CVA) promotes tissue breakdown by the following pathway:

- Stress creates drain on the adrenal glands
- Adrenaline production is increased
- Metabolism is increased
- Depletion of nutrient stores is required for healing
- Immunity is weakened
- Additional stress occurs
- Recovery is compromised and malnutrition is worsened[38]

Recommendations provided by a dietician regarding Mr. Clark's diet will be reinforced and include the following:

- Eat several small meals and take nutritional supplements
- Drink plenty of fluids throughout the day to keep blood volumes up for better delivery of oxygen to the tissues

THERAPEUTIC EXERCISE

See Neuromuscular Pattern D: Impaired Motor Function and Sensory Integrity Associated With Nonprogressive Disorders of the Central Nervous System—Acquired in Adolescence or Adulthood for exercises for this patient.

FUNCTIONAL TRAINING IN SELF-CARE AND HOME MANAGEMENT

- Self-care and home management
  - Patient should have a pressure relief support surface mattress

- In bed Mr. Clark should have his heels elevated to avoid pressure
- In bed when sidelying he should have a pillow between his knees to reduce pressure over the medial condyles of the femur
- Transfer training and pressure relief techniques during ADL should be provided to the staff and to Mr. Clark and should include:
  - Instructions in pressure relief strategies
  - Transfer training with appropriate assistive devices and use of a gait belt
- During sitting, Mr. Clark should know the proper:
  - Way to change his position for pressure relief throughout the day to avoid friction and shear on his buttocks
  - Placement of the feet and control of the pelvis to facilitate more symmetrical sitting posture

FUNCTIONAL TRAINING IN WORK, COMMUNITY, AND LEISURE INTEGRATION OR REINTEGRATION

- Work, community, and leisure
  - Transfer training and pressure relief techniques during IADL should be provided to the staff taking care of Mr. Clark and to Mr. Clark and his family

PRESCRIPTION, APPLICATION, AND, AS APPROPRIATE, FABRICATION OF DEVICES AND EQUIPMENT

- Adaptive devices
  - A pressure relief support surface mattress is indicated
  - The use of a hospital bed with pressure relief to be assessed
  - A seating system for his wheelchair is to be provided to include:
    - A pressure relief cushion that envelopes the ischial tuberosities to reduce shear and friction
- Assistive devices
  - Wheelchair
    - His wheelchair should control his pelvis and prevent sliding forward
    - His feet should be on footrests so that the thighs are parallel to the floor and the hips are in 90 degrees of flexion

INTEGUMENTARY REPAIR AND PROTECTION TECHNIQUES

- Topical agents
  - Use of a skin sealant to decrease moisture

ELECTROTHERAPEUTIC MODALITIES

♦ Electrical stimulation
  ● TENS
    ■ Conventional mode initially with short duration and high frequency
    ■ Progression to modulation mode
    ■ Instruction in TENS use also provided to the health center staff

ANTICIPATED GOALS AND EXPECTED OUTCOMES

♦ Impact on pathology/pathophysiology
  ● Nutrient delivery to tissue is increased.
  ● Pain is decreased to 1 out of 6 on the Faces Pain Scale in two treatment sessions.
♦ Impact on impairments
  ● Integumentary integrity is improved, nonblanchable erythema over the right ischial tuberosity is resolved in 2 weeks.
  ● Postural control is improved so Mr. Clark can sit more erect in his wheelchair in four treatment sessions.
  ● Shear and friction are reduced during transfers and in wheelchair
  ● Transfers are improved to minimal assistance in four treatment sessions.
♦ Impact on functional limitations
  ● Ability to perform physical actions, tasks, or activities related to self-care is improved.
  ● Caregiver ability to perform physical actions, tasks, or activities to improve and protect skin integrity is improved.
  ● Performance levels in self-care, home management, work, community, or leisure actions, tasks, or activities are improved.
  ● Tolerance to positions and activities is increased to return to playing cards with his friends at the extended care facility.
♦ Risk reduction/prevention
  ● Physical function is improved.
  ● Pressure on body tissues is reduced to acceptable levels with appropriate positioning and pressure-reducing devices.
  ● Protection of body parts is increased.
  ● Risk factors are reduced.
  ● Risk of secondary impairments is reduced.
  ● Safety is improved.
♦ Impact on health, wellness, and fitness
  ● Behaviors that foster healthy habits, wellness, and prevention are acquired.

  ● Health status is improved.
  ● Physical function is improved.
♦ Impact on societal resources
  ● Documentation occurs throughout patient management and follows APTA's *Guidelines for Physical Therapy Documentation.*[63]
  ● Referrals are made to other professionals or resources whenever necessary and appropriate.
  ● Resources area utilized in a cost-effective manner.
♦ Patient/client satisfaction
  ● Patient and family knowledge and awareness of the diagnosis, prognosis, interventions, and anticipated goals and expected outcomes are increased.
  ● Patient and family understanding of anticipated goals and expected outcomes is increased.
  ● Sense of well-being is improved.

REEXAMINATION

Reexamination is performed throughout the episode of care.

DISCHARGE

Mr. Clark is discharged from physical therapy for his integumentary impairments after a total of four sessions and attainment of his goals and expectations. These sessions have covered his entire episode of care. He is discharged because he has achieved his goals and expected outcomes.

Case Study #3: Deep Vein Thrombosis, Cellulitis, Edema

Ms. Mary Smith is a 62-year-old female with an edematous left lower extremity with cellulitis and a recent history of a deep vein thrombosis.

PHYSICAL THERAPIST EXAMINATION

HISTORY

♦ General demographics: Mary Smith is a 62-year-old black American female whose primary language is English.
♦ Social history: Ms. Smith is divorced and the mother of a son (40) and a daughter (38). She is a grandmother of two.

♦ Employment/work: Ms. Smith is a checker at the local supermarket. She has taken a medical leave due to her painful swollen leg.

♦ Living environment: She lives alone in a second floor apartment that is accessed by stairs with a railing. There is no elevator access.

♦ General health status
  • General health perception: She reports that her health status is poor.
  • Physical function: She reports that her physical function is diminished for her age.
  • Psychological function: Ms. Smith reports mild to moderate depression.
  • Role function: Store clerk, daughter, mother, and grandmother.
  • Social function: She enjoys church activities in which she now rarely participates. She currently spends the majority of her day watching television.

♦ Social/health habits: Ms. Smith is a nonsmoker and does not drink alcohol.

♦ Family history: Her mother, age 80, has diabetes and HTN. Her father died of cancer at age 65.

♦ Medical/surgical history: Ms. Smith's symptoms of edema and pain started 6 months ago when her left leg was struck with a shopping cart at the level of her ankle. She developed a DVT and was treated with anticoagulation therapy. Ms. Smith also has HTN.

♦ Current condition(s)/chief complaint(s): Ms. Smith has been informed by her physician that her DVT has resolved, but the edema and superficial erythema and new diagnosis of cellulitis persists limiting her return to her normal activities.

♦ Functional status and activity level: Ms. Smith is independent in all ADL and IADL, but due to her persistent edema, she is not able to walk for exercise.

♦ Medications: Mary is taking ibuprofen, calcium, a multivitamin, and hydrochlorothiazide (HCTZ) for HTN.

♦ Other clinical tests
  • Imaging/diagnostic tests: Venous plethysmogram was positive for left leg venous insufficiency.

SYSTEMS REVIEW

♦ Cardiovascular/pulmonary
  • BP: 145/90 mmHg
  • Edema: 3+ pitting edema of the left calf and foot
  • HR: 80 bpm
  • RR: 12 bpm

♦ Integumentary
  • Presence of scar formation: None
  • Skin color: Hyperpigmentation (brawny patches) distal LLE and ankle

  • Skin integrity: Intact but with noted trophic changes consistent with venous insufficiency including venous eczema and lipodermatosclerosis[13]

♦ Musculoskeletal
  • Gross range of motion: Limited left ankle and foot ROM
  • Gross strength: Calf muscle weaker on left when compared to right
  • Gross symmetry: Symmetrical
  • Height: 5'6" (1.68 m)
  • Weight: 175 lbs (79.38 kg)

♦ Neuromuscular
  • Transfers independent but with difficulty noted from sit to stand
  • Gait independent on level surfaces, stair climbing noted to be difficult secondary to decrease in left ankle ROM

♦ Communication, affect, cognition, language, and learning style
  • Communication, affect, cognition: Affect appeared flat but communication and cognition WFL
  • Learning preferences: Visual learner

TESTS AND MEASURES

♦ Anthropometric characteristics
  • BMI=28.12 which is higher than recommended, placing her in the overweight category
    ▪ BMI is calculated weight (175 lbs) x 700 divided by height^2 (4356 inches)
    ▪ Normal range=18.5 to 24.9
  • Edema
    ▪ 3+ pitting edema on the left from the toes to the knee
    ▪ Pitting edema may be assessed using a 1-3+ or 1-4+ scales that classify edema from minimal to severe[64,75]

♦ Assistive and adaptive devices
  • Ms. Smith uses a standard cane when she plans to be out of the house

♦ Circulation
  • Pulse exam
    ▪ Performed as an indicator of arterial blood flow
    ▪ Left DP and PT 2+ (mildly diminished)
    ▪ There are two pulse grading systems that can be incorporated (Table 2-8 and Table 3-4)[64,75]
  • Classification of CVD
    ▪ Ms. Smith is Class 4 (see Table 2-1)[14]
  • Homans' test[76]
    ▪ Is intended to identify the presence of a DVT but limited sensitivity and specificity make it a questionable test

Table 2-8	
PULSE GRADING	
0	No pulse
1+	Barely felt
2+	Diminished
3+	Easily felt
4+	Bounding

Adapted from Patterson GK. Vascular evaluation. In: Sussman C, Bates-Jensen B, eds. *Wound Care: A Collaborative Practice Manual for Physical Therapists and Nurses.* 2nd ed. Gaithersburg, Md: Aspen Publishers, Inc; 2001:178.

- Ms. Smith has limited ankle ROM and significant edema making performance of this test unsuccessful
- Ankle-brachial index (ABI)[64,75,77]
  - Is performed to indirectly assess peripheral tissue perfusion
  - ABI right was 0.8 indicating minimal to moderate ischemia
  - ABI was unable to be performed on the left due to the excessive edema
  - Interpretation of the ABI can be seen in Table 2-9[63,75]
- Cranial and peripheral nerve integrity (see Table 4-5)
  - Semmes-Weinstein monofilament testing
    - Is performed to assess sensation[64,75]
    - She is able to detect 4.17 monofilament on the plantar aspect of her left foot (indicating decreased sensation) and 5.07 on her right
- Gait, locomotion, and balance
  - Transfers independently, but with noted difficulty from sit to stand
  - Independent in ambulation with or without cane but with decreased speed
  - Able to negotiate stairs independently with her cane and railing with complaints of left ankle discomfort

- Balance is fair to good with eyes open
- Loss of balance occurs when challenged with eyes closed
- Integumentary integrity
  - Associated skin
    - Skin color
      - Erythema noted extending from left foot to 4 cm above the medial malleolus, and hemosiderosis noted in the left ankle area
      - Hemosiderosis is abnormally darker pigmentation when compared to normal skin tones usually indicating rupture of the vessels under the skin and seepage from venous HTN causing deposition of blood in the subcutaneous tissues and staining from the lysed red blood vessels[12-14]
    - Hair growth: Minimal hair noted
    - Texture: Hard and fibrotic with dry flaky skin from the midcalf to the forefoot
    - Edema: As noted above
- Muscle performance
  - Decreased strength left plantarflexion=3/5 and dorsiflexion=2/5 with given ROM
- Pain
  - Ms. Smith rates her wound pain as a 7/10 on the VAS[59-61]
- Range of motion
  - Left ankle lacks 10 degrees to neutral dorsiflexion
  - Total ROM of left ankle dorsiflexion=10 to 45 degrees
- Self-care and home management
  - Ms. Smith reports concern with the ability to don and doff compression stockings and with wearing compression stockings during the summer months
- Work, community, and leisure integration or reintegration
  - Ms. Smith also reported concern regarding her abil-

Table 2-9		
ANKLE-BRACHIAL INDEX VALUES		
ABI <0.5	Severe ischemia	Refer to vascular specialist
		Compression therapy contraindicated
ABI 0.5 to 0.8	Moderate ischemia	May be accompanied by intermittent claudication
		Refer to vascular specialist
		Compression therapy contraindicated
ABI 0.8 to 0.9	Mild ischemia	Compression therapy use with caution
ABI >1.0	Calcified vessels	Refer to vascular specialist
		Indicates calcified vessels if diabetic

Adapted from Patterson GK. Vascular evaluation. In: Sussman C, Bates-Jensen B, eds. *Wound Care: A Collaborative Practice Manual for Physical Therapists and Nurses.* 2nd ed. Gaithersburg, Md: Aspen Publishers, Inc; 2001:184.

ity to manage in her current work situation requiring prolonged standing due to her edema and pain with standing

- Use of a knee high compression stocking would allow her to return to work using her breaks for LE elevation

EVALUATION

Ms. Smith's history and risk factors previously outlined indicate that she is an black American female, nonsmoker, currently not exercising with HTN and venous insufficiency. She has impaired ankle ROM and strength that impacts proper calf muscle pumping action to promote venous return. Her venous disease classification is a 4, which indicated significant risk for extending ulceration.

DIAGNOSIS

Ms. Smith is a patient with venous insufficiency and a venous disease classification of 4 and pain. She has impaired: anthropometric characteristics; circulation; cranial and peripheral nerve integrity; gait, locomotion, and balance; integumentary integrity; muscle performance; and range of motion. She is functionally limited in self-care and home management and in work, community, and leisure actions, tasks, and activities. She is in need of supportive devices. These findings are consistent with placement in Pattern B: Impaired Integumentary Integrity Associated With Superficial Skin Involvement. These impairments, functional limitations, and supportive device needs will be addressed in determining the prognosis and the plan of care.

PROGNOSIS AND PLAN OF CARE

Over the course of the visits, the following mutually established outcomes have been determined:
- Ability to perform leisure activities is improved
- Ability to perform self-care and return to work activities is improved
- Left ankle ROM is increased
- Muscle performance is increased
- Patient/family knowledge and awareness of diagnosis, prognosis, interventions, and anticipated goals and outcomes are increased
- Risk factors (decreased physical activity) are decreased
- Risk of secondary impairment is reduced
- Skin integrity is improved

To achieve these outcomes, the appropriate interventions for this patient are determined. These will include: coordination, communication, and documentation; patient/client-related instruction; therapeutic exercise; functional training in self-care and home management; functional training in work, community, and leisure integration or reintegration; prescription, application, and, as appropriate, fabrication of devices and equipment; integumentary repair and protection techniques; and physical agents and mechanical modalities.

Based on the diagnosis and prognosis, Ms. Smith is expected to require four to six visits over a 1-month period of time. Ms. Smith is motivated to return to work and leisure activities and has good social support.

INTERVENTIONS

RATIONALE FOR SELECTED INTERVENTIONS

Therapeutic Exercise

Exercise is the choice of physical therapy interventions for individuals with balance deficits, muscle weakness, and venous insufficiency. Stick found that slow walking in normal adults reduces calf volume in a biphasic manner: a rapid decrease followed by a slow decline.[78] Impairments of joint mobility reduce the muscle-vein pump and significantly influence venous pressure physiology under both resting and activity-related conditions. Active exercise and a greater muscle mass enhance venous emptying of the healthy leg.[79] Aerobic exercise involving the LEs increases the effect of the calf muscle pump. In addition, in combination with dietary modification, aerobic exercise will assist with weight loss.

Prescription, Application, and, as Appropriate, Fabrication of Devices and Equipment

Compression therapy decreases venous HTN by supporting the superficial veins, increasing venous return through enhancement of calf muscle pump effectiveness, and decreasing peripheral edema.[80]

The compression needed at the ankle to counteract venous HTN is between 25 and 45 mmHg.[81] Patients with mild-moderate venous insufficiency without concomitant peripheral arterial disease[82] benefit from between 30 and 40 mmHg to prevent ulcer occurrence.[82-85]

Integumentary Repair and Protection Techniques

Moisturizers are generally the most effective means to address dry skin associated with trophic changes often seen in patients with venous insufficiency.[64,75]

Physical Agents and Mechanical Modalities

Compression therapy addresses wound etiology by supporting the superficial veins, enhancing calf muscle pump effectiveness, and decreasing peripheral edema. Intermittent sequential compression acts like a "milking" device to move fluid from the foot proximally. Since Ms. Smith takes diuretic medication, she should take it prior to the use of the compression pump for peak effect.[86] Vascular testing of arterial circulation indicated that compression therapy is not contraindicated due to her 2+ palpable pulses and her ABI of 0.8 on the opposite extremity. Testing of the opposite non-edematous extremity would be a valid check for arterial occlusion since testing of the opposite extremity has been found to be predictive of a like result on the affected side.[87]

COORDINATION, COMMUNICATION, AND DOCUMENTATION

Communication will occur with Ms. Smith, her family members, and other members of the health care team as she feels is appropriate. A referral to a nutritionist/dietician will be made to ensure appropriate diet for enhancing tissue repair and prevention of breakdown. All elements of the patient's management will be documented.

PATIENT/CLIENT-RELATED INSTRUCTION

The patient will be instructed in the pathology of her edema, care of her skin, the need for compression therapy, how to apply compression therapy, and a therapeutic exercise program. Because Ms. Smith is a visual learner, patient instruction will include demonstration and pictures to enhance learning and carryover of education. She will also be instructed to see a dietitian concerning her BMI.

THERAPEUTIC EXERCISE

- ♦ Flexibility exercises
  - Stretching exercises should be done after warming up, using a slow and steady stretch accompanied by deep breathing, and building hold up to 30 seconds
  - Patient instructed in general flexibility exercises for her LEs
  - An exercise handout and log book will be provided
- ♦ Gait and locomotion training
  - Gait instruction with a cane using appropriate technique will be provided for occasional use as requested by Ms. Smith
- ♦ Strength, power, and endurance training
  - Ms. Smith will be provided with an elastic band exercise program for home
  - She will be instructed to perform her exercises one to two times a day 3 to 4 days per week
  - She will be encouraged to exercise twice a day, and once she returns to work she will be encouraged to perform ankle pumps and knee bends to enhance venous flow

FUNCTIONAL TRAINING IN SELF-CARE AND HOME MANAGEMENT

- ♦ Self-care and home management
  - She will be instructed in the application of compression stockings prior to household or work activities

FUNCTIONAL TRAINING IN WORK, COMMUNITY, AND LEISURE INTEGRATION OR REINTEGRATION

- ♦ Work
  - Instruction will be given in the need for compression stockings when she returns to work as a checker at the supermarket
  - Instruction will be given in the need to perform ankle pumps throughout her work day
- ♦ Leisure
  - Ms. Smith will be encouraged to return to her church activities and walk there if possible

PRESCRIPTION, APPLICATION, AND, AS APPROPRIATE, FABRICATION OF DEVICES AND EQUIPMENT

- ♦ Supportive devices
  - Ms. Smith will be fitted for moderate compression stockings (30 to 40 mmHg)
  - She will be instructed in how to don and doff the stockings and will be provided with a wearing schedule
  - Stocking should be applied after use of the sequential compression pump and worn throughout the day

INTEGUMENTARY REPAIR AND PROTECTION TECHNIQUES

- ♦ Topical agents
  - A moisturizer to decrease the dryness noted on her LLE will be used
  - Over-the-counter moisturizers are to be applied twice a day to decrease her dry skin
  - Wound dressings are not required as the skin is intact

PHYSICAL AGENTS AND MECHANICAL MODALITIES

- ♦ Compression garments
  - Compression stockings as noted above will be utilized after the morning session of her compression therapy and throughout the day
- ♦ Compression therapies

- Vasopneumatic compression devices
  - Ms. Smith will be instructed in the use of a home compression unit
  - She should use the unit for 1 to 2 hours per day in the morning and the evening

ANTICIPATED GOALS AND EXPECTED OUTCOMES

- ◆ Impact on pathology/pathophysiology
  - Soft tissue swelling is reduced to WNL.
- ◆ Impact on impairments
  - Edema is reduced to 1+ pitting edema with activity.
  - Integumentary integrity is improved.
  - Muscle strength is improved to WFL.
  - ROM is improved to WFL.
- ◆ Impact on functional limitations
  - Ability to resume required self-care, home management, work, community, and leisure roles is improved.
  - Independence in ambulation is achieved with her cane.
  - Performance levels in self-care, home management, work, community, or leisure actions, tasks, and activities are improved
  - Tolerance to positions or activities is increased to return to prior level of function.
- ◆ Risk reduction/prevention
  - Risk factors are reduced for integumentary impairments with independent use of a compression pump to reduce edema.
  - Risk of secondary impairments is reduced.
  - Safety is improved.
  - Self-management of symptoms is improved so independent in use of compression pump.
- ◆ Impact on health, wellness, and fitness
  - Health status is improved.
  - Physical function is improved.
- ◆ Impact on societal resources
  - Documentation occurs throughout patient management and follows APTA's *Guidelines for Physical Therapy Documentation.*[63]
  - Referrals are made to other professionals or resources whenever necessary and appropriate.
  - Resources are utilized in a cost-effective manner.
- ◆ Patient/client satisfaction
  - Care is coordinated with patient/family and other professionals.
  - Patient and family understanding of anticipated goals and expected outcomes is increased.

- Patient knowledge and awareness of the diagnosis, prognosis, interventions, and anticipated goals and expected outcomes are increased.

REEXAMINATION

Reexamination is performed throughout the episode of care.

DISCHARGE

Ms. Smith is discharged from physical therapy after a total of five sessions and attainment of her goals and expectations. These sessions have covered her entire episode of care. She is discharged because she has achieved her goals and expected outcomes.

REFERENCES

1. Dykes P, Heggie R, Hill S. Effects of adhesive dressings on the stratum corneum of the skin. *Journal of Wound Care.* 2001;10(2).
2. Yosipovitch G, Hu J. The importance of skin pH. *Skin & Aging.* 2003;11:88-93.
3. Sibbald R, Cameron J. Dermatological aspects of wound care. In: Krasner D, Sibbald R, eds. *Chronic Wound Care: A Clinical Source Book for Healthcare Professionals.* 3rd ed. Wayne, Pa: HMP Communications; 2001:273-285.
4. Winter GD. Formation of the scab and the rate of epithelial-izatin of superficial wounds in the skin of the young domestic pig. *Nature.* 1962;193:293-294.
5. Little J, Kobayashi G, Bailey T. Infection of the diabetic foot. In: Levin ME, Bowker JH, eds. *The Diabetic Foot.* 5th ed. St. Louis, Mo: Mosby Year Book; 1993:181-198.
6. Halkier-Sorenson L. Understanding skin barrier dysfunction in dry skin patients. *Skin and Wound Care.* 1999;7:60-64.
7. Langemo D, Hunter S, Anderson J, Hanson D, Thompson P, Klug MG. Incorporating a body wash and skin protectant into skin care protocols reduces skin breakdown in two nursing homes. *Extended Care Products News.* 2003:36-37.
8. Eaglstein W. Wound healing and aging. *Clin Geriatr Med.* 1989;5(1):183-188.
9. Ashcroft G, Horan M, Herrick SE, Tarnuzzer RW, Schultz GS, Ferguson MW. Age-related differences in the temporal and spatial regulation of matrix metalloproteinases (MMPs) in normal skin and acute cutaneous wounds of healthy humans. *Cell & Tissue Research.* 1997;290(3):581-591.
10. Sussman C, Bates-Jensen B. Wound healing physiology and chronic wound healing. In: Sussman C, Bates-Jensen B, eds. *Wound Care: A Collaborative Practice Manual for Physical Therapists and Nurses.* 2nd ed. Gaithersburg, Md: Aspen; 2001:26-48.
11. Jelinek JE. Dermatology. In: Levin M, Bowker JH, eds. *The Diabetic Foot.* 5th ed. St. Louis, Mo: Mosby Year Book; 1993:61-77.
12. Hurley J. Chronic venous insufficiency: venous ulcers and other consequences. In: Krasner D, ed. *Chronic Wound Care:*

A Clinical Source Book for Health Care Professionals. 1st ed. Wayne, Pa: Health Management Publications, Inc; 1990:213-222.

13. Geyer M, Brienza D, Chib V, Wang J. Quantifying fibrosis in venous disease: mechanical properties of lipodermatosclerotic and healthy tissue. *Advances in Skin and Wound Care.* 2004;17:131-141.

14. Kistner R, Eklof B, Masuda E. Diagnosis of chronic venous disease of the lower extremities: the "CEAP" classification. *Mayo Clin Proc.* 1996;71(4):338-345.

15. Carpentier P, Cornu-Thenard A, Uhl J, Partsch H, Antignani P, Societe Francaise de Medicine Vascularie; European Working Group on the Clinical Characterization of Venous Disorders. Appraisal of the information content of the C classes of CEAP clinical classification of chronic venous disorders: a multicenter evaluation of 872 patients. *Journal of Vascular Surgery.* 2003;37(4):827-833.

16. Greene D, Feldman E, Stevens M. Neuropathy in the diabetic foot: new concepts in etiology and treatment. In: Levin ME, Bowker JH, ed. *The Diabetic Foot.* 5th ed. St. Louis, Mo: Mosby Year Book; 1993:135-148.

17. Levin ME. Pathogenesis and management of diabetic foot lesions. In: Levin ME, Bowker JH, ed. *The Diabetic Foot.* 5th ed. St. Louis, Mo: Mosby Year Book; 1993:17-60.

18. Jude E, Armstrong D, Boulton AJM. Assessment of the diabetic foot. In: Krasner D, Sibbald R, eds. *Chronic Wound Care: A Clinical Source Book for Healthcare Professionals.* 3rd ed. Wayne, Pa: HMP Communications; 2001:591-597.

19. Bernstein RK. Physical signs of the intrinsic minus foot. *Diabetes Care.* 2003;26(4):1945.

20. Bus S, Yang Q, Wang J, Smith M, Wunderlich R, Cavanagh P. Intrinsic muscle atrophy and toe deformity in the diabetic neuropathic foot: a magnetic resonance imaging study. *Diabetes Care.* 2002;25(8):1444-1450.

21. Sinacore DR, Muller M, J. Pedal ulcers in older adults with diabetes mellitus. *Topics in Geriatric Rehabilitation.* 2000;16(2):11-23.

22. McMillan DE. Hemorheology. In: Levin ME, Bowker JH, eds. *The Diabetic Foot.* 5th ed. St. Louis, Mo: Mosby Year Book; 1993:115-133.

23. Smith RG. Validation of Wagner's classification: a literature review. *Ostomy/Wound Management.* 2003;49(1):54-62.

24. Wagner FEW. The dysvascular foot: a system for diagnosis and treatment. *Foot and Ankle.* 1981;(2):64-122.

25. Armstrong D, Lavery L, Harkless L. Validation of a diabetic wound classification system. The contribution of depth, infection, and ischemia to risk of amputation. *Diabetes Care.* 1998;21(5):855-859.

26. Teasell R, Malcolm J, Arnold O, Krassioukov A, Delaney G. Cardiovascular consequences of loss of supraspinal control of the sympathetic nervous system after spinal cord injury. *Arch Phys Med Rehabil.* 2000;81(4):506-516.

27. Maklebust J, Sieggreen M. Etiology and pathophysiology of pressure ulcers. In: Maklebust J, Sieggreen M, eds. *Pressure Ulcers: Guidelines for Prevention and Nursing Management.* 1st ed. West Dundee, Ill: SN Publications; 1991:19-27.

28. Stotts N, Wipke-Tevis D. Co-factors in impaired wound healing. In: Krasner D, Kane D, eds. *Chronic Wound Care: A Clinical Sourcebook for Health Care Professionals.* 2nd ed. Wayne, Pa: Health Management Publications, Inc; 1997:64-71.

29. Chidester J, Spangler A. Fluid intake in the institutionalized elderly. *J Am Diet Assoc.* 1997;97:23-28.

30. Consultant Dieticians in Health Care Facilities. *Pocket Resource for Nutrition Assessment Rev.* The American Dietetic Association; 2001.

31. Childester J, Spanger AA. Fluid intake in the institutional elderly. *J Am Diet Assoc.* 1997;9:23-28.

32. Bernstein L, Bachman TE, Meguid M, et al. Measurement of visceral protein status in assessing protein and energy malnutrition: standard of care. Prealbumin in Nutritional Care Consensus Group. *Nutrition.* 1995;11:170.

33. Posthaur ME. Nutritional assessment and treatment. In: Sussman C, Bates-Jensen BM, ed. *Wound Care: A Collaborative Practice Manual for Physical Therapists and Nurses.* 2nd ed. Gaithersburg, Md: Aspen; 2001:52-76.

34. Marston W, Carlin R, Passman M, Farber M, Keegy B. Healing rates and cost efficacy of outpatient compression treatment for leg ulcers associated with venous insufficiency. *Journal of Vascular Surgery.* 1999;30(3):491-498.

35. Belcher AE. Skin care for the oncology patient. In: Krasner D, Kane D, eds. *Chronic Wound Care: A Clinical Sourcebook for Health Care Professionals.* Vol 1. 2nd ed. Wayne, Pa: Health Management Publications, Inc; 1997:64-71.

36. Braden B. The relationship between stress and pressure sore formation. *Ostomy/Wound Management.* 1998;44(3A Suppl):26S-36S.

37. Cole-King A, Harding K. Psychological factors and delayed healing in chronic wounds. *Psychosom Med.* 2001;63:216-220.

38. Cataldo C, DeBruyne L, Whitney E. *Nutrition and Diet Therapy.* Belmont, Calif: Wadsworth Group, Division of Thomson Learning; 1999.

39. Wound Ostomy CNS. Indentifying and treating reversible causes of urinary incontinence. *Ostomy/Wound Management.* 2003;49(12):28-33.

40. Aly R. Microbial infections of skin and nails. In: Baron S, ed. *Medical Microbiology.* 4th ed. Galveston, Tex: The University of Texas Medical Branch at Galveston; 1996:1159-1168. Online edition retrieved from http://GSBS.UTMB.edu/microbook/ch1198.htm.

41. Sibbald RG. Topical antimicrobials. *Ostomy/Wound Management.* 2003;49(5A):14-18.

42. Bergstrom N, Allman RM, Carlson CE, et al. *Pressure Ulcers in Adults: Prediction and Preventions.* Rockville, Md: US Dept of Health and Human Services; May 1992:3.

43. Bergstrom N, Allman RM, Alvarez OM, Bennet MA, Carlson CE, Frantz R. Clinical Practice Guideline: Treatment of Pressure Ulcers. Rockville MD: Us Department of Health and Human Services, Public Health Service, Agency for Health Care Policy and Research; 1994:15.

44. Maklebust J, Sieggreen M. In: Maklebust J, Sieggreen M, eds. *Pressure Ulcers: Guidelines for Prevention and Nursing Management.* West Dundee, Ill: SN Publications; 1991:24.

45. Henderson C, Ayello C, Sussman C. Draft definition of stage I pressure ulcers: inclusion of person with darkly pigmented skin. *Advances in Skin and Wound Care.* 1997;10:34-35.

46. National Pressure Ulcer Advisory Panel. Pressure ulcers, prevalence, cost, and risk assessment: consensus development conference statement. *Decubitus.* 1989;2(2):24-28.

47. Knuutinen. Smoking effects collagen synthesis and extra-celllular matrix turnover in human skin. *Br J Dermatol.*

2002;146(4):588-594.

48. Sibbald R, Williamson D, Orsted H. Preparing the wound bed: debridement, bacterial balance, and moisture balance. *Ostomy/Wound Management*. 2000;46(11):14-35.

49. Lewis CD. Peripheral arterial disease of the lower extremity. *J Cardiovasc Nurs*. 2001;15(4):45-63.

50. Blank CA, Irwin GH. Peripheral vascular disorders: assessment and intervention. *Nurs Clin North Am*. 1990;25(4):777-794.

51. Ward K, Schwartz ML, Thiele R, Yoon P. Lower extremity manifestations of vascular disease. *Clin Podiatr Med Surg*. 1998;15(4):629-672.

52. Schriger D, Baraff L. Defining normal capillary refill: variation with age, sex, and temperature. *Ann Emerg Med*. 1988;17(9):932-935.

53. Strozik K, Pieper C, Cools F. Capillary refill time in newborns: optimal pressing time, site of testing and normal values. *Acta Paediatr*. 1998;87(3):310-312.

54. Bates-Jensen BM. Chronic wound assessment. *Nurs Clin North Am*. 1999;34(4):799-845.

55. Gorelick MH, Shaw KN, Murphy KO. Validity and reliability of clinical signs in the diagnosis of dehydration in children. *Pediatrics*. 1997;99(5):e6.

56. Collins KA, Sumpio BE. Vascular assessment. *Clin Podiatr Med Surg*. 2000;17(2):171-191.

57. McGee SR, Boyko EJ. Physical examination and chronic lower-extremity ischemia: a critical review. *Arch Intern Med*. 1998;158:1357-1364.

58. Doughty DB, Waldrop J, Ramundo J. Lower-extremity ulcers of vascular etiology. In: Bryant RA, ed. *Acute and Chronic Wounds: Nursing Management*. St. Louis, Mo: Mosby; 2000.

59. Ferraz M, Quaresma M, Aquino L, Atra E, Tugwell P, Goldsmith C. Reliability of pain scales in the assessment of literate and illiterate patients with rheumatoid arthritis. *J Rheumatol*. 1990;17(8):1022-1024.

60. Hoher J, Munster A, Klein J, Eypasch E, Tilling T. Validation and application of a subjective knee questionnaire. *Knee Surg Sports Traumatol Arthrosc*. 1995;3(1):26-33.

61. Paice JA, Cohen FL. Validity of a verbally administered numeric rating scale to measure cancer pain intensity. *Cancer Nurs*. 1997;20(2):88-93.

62. Wachtel TL, Berry CC, Wachtel EE, Frank HA. The inter-rater reliability of estimating the size of burns from various burn area chart drawings. *Burns*. 2000;26(2):156-170.

63. American Physical Therapy Association. *Guide to Physical Therapist Practice*. 2nd ed. Alexandria, Va: American Physical Therapy Association; 2001.

64. Myers BA. *Wound Management: Principles and Practice*. Upper Saddle River, NJ: Prentice Hall; 2004.

65. Richard R. Assessment and diagnosis of burn wounds. *Advances in Skin and Wound Care*. 1999;12(9):468-471.

66. Burgess MC. Initial management of a patient with extensive burn injury. *Crit Care Nurs North Am*. 1991;3(2):165-179.

67. Braden B. Assessment in pressure ulcer prevention. In: Krasner D, ed. *Chronic Wound Cares*. 3rd ed. Wayne, Pa: Health Management Publications, Inc; 2001:641-651.

68. Examples of pain intensity scales for use with older patients. *Pain*. 1990;41:139-150.

69. Cosmo P, Svensson H, Brommy S, So W. Effect of transcutaneous nerve stimulation on the microcirculation in chronic leg ulcers. *Scand J Plast Reconstr Surg Hand Surg*. 2000;34(Mar):61-64.

70. Cramp A, Gilsensan C, Lowe A, Walsh D. The effect of high and low frequency transcutaneous electrical nerve stimulation upon cutaneous blood flow and skin temperature in healthy subjects. *Clin Physiol*. 2000;20(2):150-157.

71. Forst T, Pfutzner A, Bauersachs R, et al. Comparison of the microvascular response to transcutaneous electrical nerve stimulation and post occlusive ischemia in the diabetic foot. *J Diabetes Complications*. 1997;11(5):291-297.

72. Wikstrom S, Svedman P, Svensson H, Tanweer H. Effecct of transcutaneous nerve stimulation on microcirculation in intact skin and blister wounds in healthy volunteers. *Scand J Plast Reconstr Surg Hand Surg*. 1999;33(2):195-201.

73. Kumar D, Alvaro MS, Julka IS, Marshall HJ. Diabetic peripheral neuropathy effectiveness of electrotherapy and amitriptyline for symptomatic relief. *Diabetes Care*. 1998;21(8):1322-1325.

74. Julka IS, Alvaro MS, Kumar D. Beneficial effects of electrical stimulation on neuropathis symptoms in diabetes patients. *J Foot Ankle Surg*. 1998;37(3):191-193.

75. Sussman C, Bates-Jensen BM, eds. *Wound Care: A Collaborative Practice Manual for Physical Therapists and Nurses*. Gaithersburg, Md: Aspen Publishers, Inc; 1998.

76. Wells PS, Hirsh J, Anderson DR, et al. Accuracy of clinical assessment of deep-vein thrombosis. *Lancet*. 1995;345(8961):1326-1330.

77. Kloth LC, McCulloch JM. *Wound Healing Alternatives in Management*. 3rd ed. Philadelphia, Pa: FA Davis Co; 2002.

78. Stick C, Jaeger H, Witzleb E. Measurement of volume changes and venous pressure in the human lower leg during walking and running. *J Appl Physiol*. 1992;72(6):2063-2068.

79. Kugler C, Strunk M, Rudofsky G. Venous pressure dynamics of the healthy human leg: role of muscle activity, joint mobility and anthropometric factors. *J Vasc Res*. 2001;38(1):20-29.

80. Moore Z. Compression bandaging: are practitioners achieving the ideal sub-bandage pressures? *J Wound Care*. 2002;11(7):265-268.

81. Bryant L. Management of edema. In: Sussman C, Bates-Jensen B, eds. *Wound Care: A Collaborative Practice Manual for Physical Therapists and Nurses*. 2nd ed. Gaithersburg, Md: Aspen Publishers, Inc; 2001:235-255.

82. McGuckin M, Williams L, Brooks J, Cherry GW. Guidelines in practice: the effect on healing of venous ulcers. *Advances in Skin and Wound Care*. 2001;14(1):33-36.

83. Cullum N, Nelson E, Fletcher AW, Sheldon TA. Compression for venous leg ulcers (Cochrane Review). *The Cochrane Library (2)*. 2002.

84. Bergan JJ, Sparks SR. Non-elastic compression: an alternative in management of chronic venous insufficiency. *J Wound Ostomy Continence Nurs*. 2000;27(2):83-89.

85. Nelson E, Bell-Syer S, et al. Compression for preventing recurrence of venous ulcers. *The Cochrane Library (2)*. 2000.

86. Kugler SM, Rudofsky G. Venous pressure dynamics of the healthy human leg: role of muscle activity, joint mobility and anthropometric factors. *J Vasc Res*. 2001;38(1):20-29.

87. Kazmers KM, Broehn H, Oust G, et al. Assessment of noninvasive lower extremity arterial testing versus pulse exam. *Am Surg*. 1996;62(4):315-319.

Color Atlas

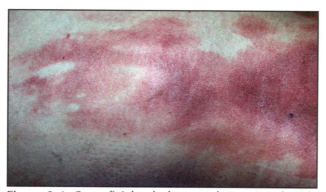

Figure 2-1. Superficial splash wound. Reprinted with permission from Myers B. *Wound Management: Principles and Practice.* East Rutherford, NJ: Pearson Education; 2003. (Please see original figure on page 25.)

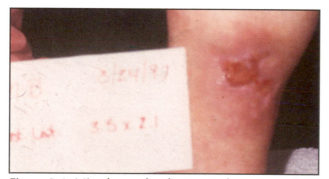

Figure 3-1. Mixed vascular disease and pressure ulcer. (Please see original figure on page 54.)

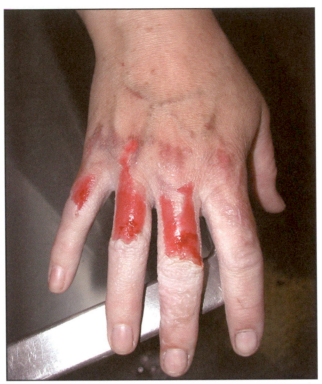

Figure 3-2. Superficial partial-thickness burn wound. (Please see original figure on page 61.)

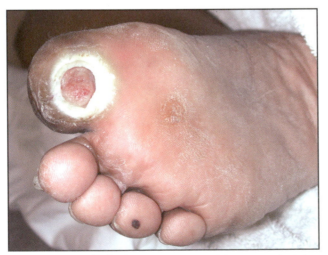

Figure 4-2. Full-thickness neuropathic wound right great toe. (Please see original figure on page 77.)

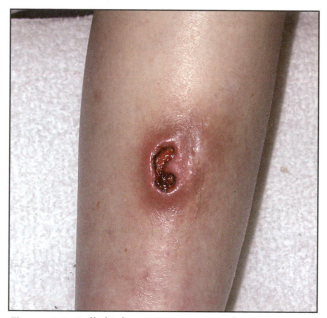

Figure 4-3. Full-thickness traumatic and arterial insufficiency wound right anterior lower leg. (Please see original figure on page 83.)

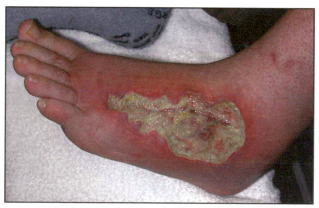

Figure 4-4. Full-thickness infected wound on the dorsal aspect of the left foot. (Please see original figure on page 89.)

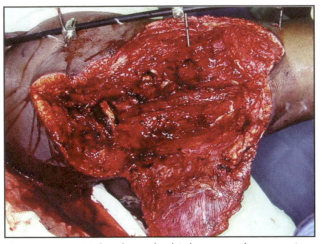

Figure 5-1. Right lateral thigh wound operative debridement and external fixator placement. (Please see original figure on page 106.)

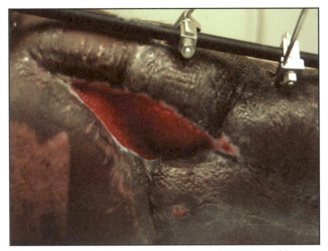

Figure 5-2. Right lateral thigh wound at time of home discharge. (Please see original figure on page 111.)

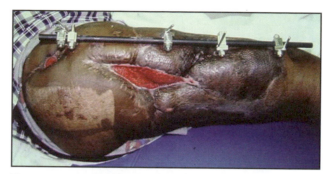

Figure 5-3. Right lateral thigh wound at time of 6-week follow-up appointment with MD. (Please see original figure on page 112.)

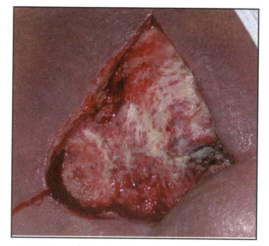

Figure 5-4. Sacral wound at time of initial physical therapy examination. (Please see original figure on page 113.)

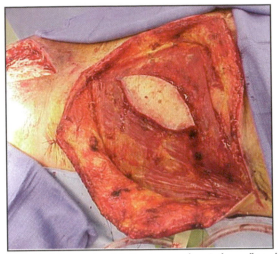

Figure 5-5. Harvest of latissimus dorsi free flap by plastic surgeon. (Please see original figure on page 117.)

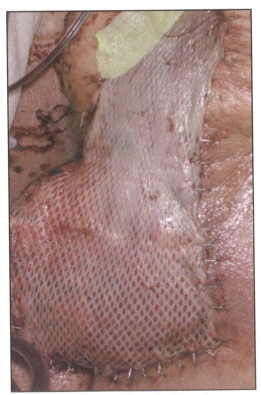

Figure 5-6. Sacral wound with free flap coverage. (Please see original figure on page 118.)

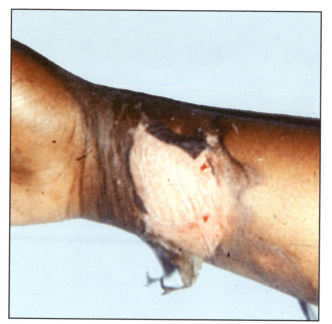

Figure 5-7. Right wrist high-volt electrical injury. (Please see original figure on page 120.)

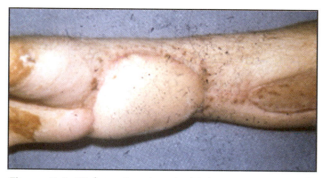

Figure 5-8. Right wrist electrical injury approximately 4 months post musculocutaneous free flap. (Please see original figure on page 122.)

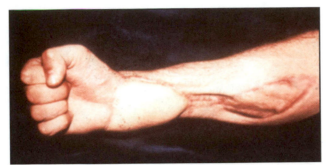

Figure 5-9. Right wrist electrical injury 1 year post injury. (Please see original figure on page 123.)

Impaired Integumentary Integrity Associated With Partial-Thickness Skin Involvement and Scar Formation (Pattern C)

Betsy A. Myers, PT, MPT, MHS, OCS, CLT

INTRODUCTION

Partial-thickness wounds involve the epidermis and part of the dermis. Examples of partial-thickness wounds include Stage II pressure ulcers (see Table 2-7), Wagner Grade 1 (see Table 2-2) neuropathic ulcers, superficial and deep partial-thickness (or second-degree) burns, as well as some ulcers due to vascular insufficiency, trauma, or surgery. Although vascular insufficiency ulcers may range from superficial skin involvement (Pattern B: Impaired Integumentary Integrity Associated With Superficial Skin Involvement) to full-thickness extending into fascia, muscle, or bone (Pattern E: Impaired Integumentary Integrity Associated With Skin Involvement Extending Into Fascia, Muscle, or Bone and Scar Formation), the majority of these ulcers that require physical therapy interventions will have partial (Pattern C: Impaired Integumentary Integrity Associated With Partial-Thickness Skin Involvement and Scar Formation) or full-thickness (Pattern D: Impaired Integumentary Integrity Associated With Full-Thickness Skin Involvement and Scar Formation) skin involvement.[1,2]

ANATOMY

The anatomy of the skin has been reviewed in Pattern A: Primary Prevention/Risk Reduction for Integumentary Disorders. Since the majority of ulcers in this pattern are the result of vascular insufficiency, the anatomy will concentrate on the vascular system. The cardiovascular system delivers oxygen and nutrients to body cells and removes waste products. It is comprised of the heart, arteries, capillaries, and veins. The arterial system is the high-pressure system that carries blood from the left ventricle to the body's tissues. Arteries have three layers: the adventitia, tunica media, and tunica intima.[3] The adventitia is the outer layer that provides protection and support for the vessel. The tunica media is the muscular middle layer. This layer is innervated by the sympathetic nervous system, allowing the modulation of vessel lumen size, either vasoconstriction or vasodilation, based on tissue demands.[4] The inner tunica intima is comprised of a thin layer of endothelial cells that are in direct contact with circulating blood. The tunica intima is thin and fragile, making it easily traumatized.[5] Blood moves from the arterioles into the capillaries, 1-mm-long vessels composed of a single layer of endothelial cells and a thin basement membrane. The capillary lumen is wide enough for only a single layer of red blood cells to pass through.[4]

Blood moves from the capillaries into the veins. Like arteries, veins are comprised of three layers: adventitia, tunica media, and intimal layer.[3,6,7] However, because these layers are thinner and contain less connective tissue and muscular support, veins are more extensible and can accommodate a larger volume of blood than arteries. There are three main types of veins.[8] The deep veins, including the femoral, popliteal, and tibial veins, are located within the muscles roughly paralleling arteries of the same names. The superficial veins, including the greater and lesser saphenous veins, are housed within the subcutaneous tissues. Short, perforating veins connect the two networks allowing blood to flow from the superficial to the deep veins. Veins are divided into short segments by a series of bicuspid valves.[8,9]

PHYSIOLOGY

Blood is propelled into the arterial system by powerful contractions of the left ventricle. BP within the proximal segments of the arterial system is generally 90 to 100 mmHg and will decrease to 25 to 35 mmHg within the smaller, more distal arterioles. Pressure decreases approximately 10 mmHg as blood travels through the thin, narrow capillaries. Within the capillaries, oxygen and nutrients diffuse across the capillary membrane along their concentration gradients into the tissues while carbon dioxide and metabolic wastes diffuse in the opposite direction.[4] BP within the venous system plummets from approximately 15 mmHg at the vein-capillary junction to almost 0 mmHg upon reaching the right atrium.[10]

Blood flows through this low-pressure system, primarily against gravity and without the benefit of the powerful left atrium, and is assisted in three ways. First, the bicuspid valves within the veins allow blood to flow in only one direction, proximally, toward the heart.[8,9] Second, when the muscles surrounding the deep veins (specifically the gastrocnemius and soleus in the lower leg) contract, they increase the pressure within the deep veins, forcing blood to move proximally.[6,11,12] The calf muscle pump is particularly important within the LE where intermittent contraction and relaxation of the gastrocnemius-soleus complex during walking helps propel blood against gravity up the leg, while intact valves prevent retrograde, gravity-assisted venous blood flow.[13] Third, proximally directed venous blood flow is assisted by the alternating pressures created during breathing.[10,14] Pressure changes within the thorax create this respiratory pump. As the diaphragm descends during inspiration, the pressure within the thoracic cavity is decreased while there is a concomitant increase in abdominal pressure. This pressure gradient forces blood to flow proximally toward the right atrium. The greater the inspiration, the greater the pressure gradient and the greater the assist of proximally directed venous blood flow.

PATHOPHYSIOLOGY

ARTERIAL INSUFFICIENCY

Arterial ulcers are caused by a critical decrease in arterial blood flow, also known as arterial insufficiency. Five to 10%

of all LE ulcers and 5% of all amputations are due to arterial insufficiency.[15] Although there are many possible causes of arterial insufficiency, including trauma, acute embolism, and Buerger's disease, the primary cause is the thickening and hardening of arterial walls, generally referred to as arteriosclerosis.[16] The most common form of arteriosclerosis within the United States is atherosclerosis, a systemic degenerative process whereby cholesterol is deposited within vessel walls forming fatty streaks or plaques. Cholesterol deposition promotes vessel stenosis directly because these plaques grow, causing progressive narrowing of the vessel lumen. In addition, cholesterol deposition indirectly leads to vessel stenosis by triggering biochemical changes and intimal cell injury.[17] When the body attempts to repair damaged endothelial cells, there is a build-up of platelets and fibrous scarring that encroaches upon the vessel lumen. Atherosclerosis is also thought to cause thickening of the capillary basement membrane,[5] decreasing diffusion of oxygen and nutrients to the tissues. Risk factors for arteriosclerosis are hyperlipidemia, elevated low-density lipoproteins, smoking, diabetes, HTN, trauma, and advanced age.[18,19] By controlling modifiable risk factors, the development and progression of arteriosclerosis may be reduced.

Patients with mild atherosclerosis may not have any overt symptoms. As vessel stenosis progresses, patients may complain of intermittent claudication, activity-specific discomfort due to local tissue ischemia.[20] As stenosis continues to progress the existing blood supply may no longer be able to meet the basic metabolic tissue demands, leading to ischemic rest pain. It is possible for patients to develop spontaneous ulcerations due to arterial insufficiency. However, the more likely cause of arterial insufficiency ulcers is a relatively minor trauma, such as a blister, abrasion, or skin tear, to an already poorly perfused limb.[17,21] Although there may be enough oxygen to maintain tissue integrity, the added metabolic demands required for tissue repair and regeneration exceeds the available supply of oxygen and nutrients, resulting in skin breakdown.[22]

Because arterial insufficiency can result in variable amounts of tissue ischemia, pain may result. Patients with suspected vascular insufficiency should be asked specifically about pain modulation with various positions and activities. The pain of arterial insufficiency is generally quite significant and increases with activities that increase tissue oxygen demands, such as ambulation.[17] Patients with arterial insufficiency ulcers generally report increased pain in positions that further impair arterial blood flow, such as LE elevation.[23] If severe, even the gravity-lessened position of laying flat supine may produce or exacerbate the pain of arterial insufficiency.

Ulcers due to arterial insufficiency have some characteristic features. First, they are almost always located in the distal LEs including the tips of the toes, dorsum of the foot, lateral malleolus, and areas of sustained trauma. This is due to the distance the blood must travel to reach these locations. Second, they generally begin as small, shallow wounds that gradually increase in size. Third, the wound bed is typically dry with significant amounts of necrotic tissue. Granulation tissue, if present, is pale due to ischemia. Gangrene may be present in severe cases.[17] Fourth, trophic changes, such as loss of hair follicles, thinning of the epidermis, and nail fungal infections, are common.[24] The limb may appear pale or dusky and is likely to be cool to the touch.

VENOUS INSUFFICIENCY

Venous insufficiency ulcers are caused by the hypoxic environment created by venous HTN.[11,25] The two main cases for venous HTN, and hence venous insufficiency ulcerations, are vein dysfunction and calf muscle pump failure.[26] Vein valves become incompetent if they fail to close completely, allowing retrograde venous blood flow and venous HTN. Degeneration, direct trauma, or scarring after tissue repair or previous thrombosis may lead to valve dysfunction. In addition, an inherent weakness in the vein walls, or varicosity, may prevent normally functioning valve flaps from approximating, leading to an increase in venous back pressure. Recall that the calf muscle pump creates pressure gradients that, along with competent vein valves, help propel venous blood toward the heart. Calf muscle pump effectiveness can be decreased by calf muscle weakness or inhibited ankle mobility due to pain, joint dysfunction, or immobilization.[7] Patients who are at risk for venous insufficiency ulcers include those individuals with vein dysfunction, calf muscle pump impairment, advanced age,[6] or a history of diabetes.[25,27] In addition, patients with a prior history of venous insufficiency ulcers are at increased risk of reulceration.[2,28]

One to 2% of the population has been diagnosed with chronic venous insufficiency,[26,29] and a significant portion of those with chronic venous insufficiency will develop an ulceration.[6] Seventy to 90% of all LE ulcers are due to chronic venous insufficiency.[6,26,30] There are two theories as to why venous insufficiency ulcers occur.[31] According to the fibrin cuff theory, venous HTN and distension lead to increased vessel permeability. Fluid and proteins move from within the veins to the interstitium causing peripheral edema. Within the tissues, the protein fibrinogen is converted into fibrin. The fibrin then adheres to capillary walls, forming a "cuff" or barrier to the normal diffusion of oxygen and nutrients.[13,32] Alternatively, the white blood cell trapping theory proposes that venous HTN and distension cause congestion. As blood flow is decreased within affected veins and their capillary networks, white blood cells begin to marginate and eventually adhere to vessel walls. The now "trapped" cells create a physical barrier to circulation. Additionally, these white blood cells migrate into the interstitium where they release proteolytic enzymes, free radicals,

and other inflammatory substances, further contributing to endothelial cell damage. According to the white blood cell trapping theory, ulceration results from local tissue hypoxia due to venous congestion, white blood cell trapping, and the increased tissue demands caused by the ensuing inflammatory response.[13] Venous insufficiency ulcers are likely the result of a combination of white blood cell trapping and fibrin cuff development.[22]

In contrast to the ischemic pain of arterial insufficiency, the pain of venous insufficiency is due to venous HTN and the resulting edema. Therefore, these patients generally report more of a dull, aching pain.[1] Patients generally report that the pain decreases with positions or interventions that increase venous return, such as elevation[33] or compression.[6] Conversely, positions that exacerbate venous HTN, such as dependency, will generally increase patient discomfort.

Ulcers due to venous insufficiency have some characteristic features. First, they are most frequently found on the medial aspect of the lower leg superior to the malleolus. Second, they have moderate to high amounts of drainage. The periwound may appear macerated if the dressing is unable to absorb this fluid. Third, the wound bed contains granular tissue but may have a thin, yellow, fibrous coating making it appear glossy. Fourth, typical skin changes include the dark brown skin staining of hemosiderin deposition as well as cellulitis. Fifth, superficial varicosities and lower leg/foot edema are the norm. The leg may be warm to touch. Table 3-1 details the typical characteristics of vascular insufficiency ulcers.

MIXED VASCULAR DISEASE

An estimated 10% to 15% of all LE ulcerations are due to impaired tissue oxygenation resulting from a combination of both arterial and venous insufficiency.[6,9,25] The presentation of patients with mixed vascular disease is quite variable and is dependent upon which system, arterial or venous, is more impaired. For example, a patient with mild arterial insufficiency and moderate to severe venous insufficiency may find pain relief from elevation and dependency but increased pain with compression (due to a further reduction in arterial flow) and ambulation (due to increased oxygen demand from working muscles). Similarly, wound bed presentation of mixed vascular insufficiency ulcers will also be quite variable.

IMAGING

The following imaging techniques and special tests may be utilized to assess circulation or tissue oxygenation.
♦ Arteriography/venography[7,24,34-37]
  • Are the most accurate methods of assessing local and regional blood flow in an extremity
  • During this procedure, a radiopaque dye is injected

Table 3-1

TYPICAL CHARACTERISTICS OF VASCULAR INSUFFICIENCY ULCERS

Characteristic	Aterial Insufficiency Ulcer	Venous Insufficiency Ulcer
Pain	May be significant	Mild
	Increased with elevation, ambulation, and compression	Decreased with elevation, ambulation, and compression
	Decreased with dependency	Increased with dependency
Location	Distal LE	Superior to medial malleolus
	Areas of trauma	Areas of trauma
Wound Bed	Dry, necrotic tissue	Granular, glossy, moderate drainage
Other	Hair loss, thinning epidermis	Hemosiderin deposition
	Pale, cool	Edema, superficial varicosities
		Warm

into the artery or vein to provide a radiographic image of blood flow

- Venogram is 100% sensitive and 100% specific for identifying deep vein thrombosis[38]
- Magnetic resonance angiography (MRA)[20,39,40]
  - Is a sensitive, reliable, accurate method of determining vessel stenosis
    - 98.6% sensitive, 100% specific, 100% positive predictive value, 99% negative predictive value, 100% concordant with angiography findings
  - Uses non-nephrotoxic contrast agent
- Digital plethysmography[26,35,41]
  - Is a noninvasive method of assessing regional blood flow to an extremity (Table 3-2)
  - Assesses the degree of valve insufficiency and calf muscle efficiency
  - More accurate than duplex imaging for infrapatellar vessels[24]
- Transcutaneous oxygen measurements (tcpO$_2$)[17,34,35,42]
  - Is used to assess oxygen tension within periwound tissues and assist with determining the most appropriate plan of care (Table 3-3)
- Color duplex ultrasonagraphy[17,20,35-37,43]
  - Is a noninvasive alternative to arteriography utilizing Doppler waveform and real-time imaging
  - Safe, low cost, rapid results[38]
  - Provides information on vessel structure, direction of blood flow, blood velocity, and turbulence of blood flow
  - Gold standard for identifying presence of deep vein thrombosis in the femoral and popliteal veins
  - Provides most accuracy in suprapatellar vessels[24]

PHARMACOLOGY

The following pharmacological agents may be utilized in the management of patients with peripheral vascular disease.

- Antihypertensive agents[44,45]
  - Diuretics
    - Examples: Bendroflumethiazide, benzthiazide, chlorothiazide, cyclothiazide, furosemide, bumetanide
    - Actions: Increase urine formation, increase sodium excretion, and decrease peripheral vascular resistance
    - Administered: Oral or parenteral
    - Side effects: Fluid depletion, electrolyte imbalance, gastrointestinal disturbances, orthostatic hypotension
  - Beta-blockers
    - Examples: Propranolol, metoprolol, atenolol
    - Actions: Lower BP by decreasing cardiac output, HR, and stroke volume by competing with catecholamines at beta-adrenergic receptors
    - Administered: Oral or parenteral
    - Side effects: Bronchoconstriction, depression of HR and myocardial contraction, orthostatic hypotension
  - Calcium channel blockers
    - Examples: Verapamil, diltiazem HCl
    - Actions: Inhibit calcium influx into arterial smooth muscle thereby decreasing vasoconstriction
    - Administered: Oral or parenteral
    - Side effects: Peripheral edema, orthostatic hypotension, abnormalities in HR
  - Angiotensin converting enzyme (ACE) inhibitors
    - Examples: Captopril, benazepril, enalapril

Table 3-2	
DIGITAL PLETHYSMOGRAPHY	
Purpose	Noninvasive method of assessing regional blood flow to an extremity
Method	A specialized cuff connected to a force transducer is placed around the extremity or digit to be assessed
	The pulsatile nature of blood flow produces pressure changes that are identified by the force transducer and graphically recorded
Interpretation	Graph provides information about blood flow, velocity, and turbulence within both arteries and veins
Advantages	Because this test records volume changes, it is more accurate than an ABI, especially in the presence of vessel calcification
Limitations	Requires specialized equipment

Table 3-3	
TRANSCUTANEOUS OXYGEN MEASUREMENTS	
Purpose	To assess oxygen tension within periwound tissues and assist with determining the most appropriate plan of care
Method	With the patient lying comfortably supine, a series of sensors are placed adjacent to the wound
	If an extremity is being tested, sensors may also be placed more proximally along the patient's extremity
Interpretation	50 mmHg=Normal tissue oxygen levels
	35 mmHg=Sufficient to support normal wound healing
	<30 mmHg=Unlikely to heal without surgical interventions, such as revascularization
Advantages	Helpful in determining appropriate plan of care such as the need for adjunctive interventions (electrotherapeutic modalities) or revascularization
	Valid and reliable measure
Limitations	Requires specialized equipment
	Costly to perform

- Actions: Decrease vasoconstriction by inhibiting conversion of angiotensin I to angiotensin II
- Administered: Oral or parenteral
- Side effects: Persistent dry cough
- Centrally acting sympatholytic drugs[25]
  - Example: Clonidine
  - Actions: Decrease vasomotor tone and peripheral vascular resistance, decrease HR and cardiac output
  - Administered: Oral or parenteral
  - Side effects: Dry mouth, dizziness, sedation
- Hemorrheologic agents
  - Cilostazol
    - Actions: A phosphodiesterase inhibitor with antiplatelet, vasodilatory, and lipid altering effects[20,46]
  - Pentoxifylline
    - Actions: Enhances local tissue perfusion; proposed methods of action include decreasing blood viscosity, decreasing platelet aggregation, and increasing red blood cell flexibility[20,31,34,47-52]
- Dalteparin
  - Actions: An antithrombolytic and anti-inflammatory that has been shown to enhance wound healing in patients with arterial insufficiency and diabetes most likely by enhancing microcirculation[53]
- Transdermal nitroglycerin patches
  - Actions: Inhibit platelet aggregation and cause local vasodilation by relaxing smooth muscles[44]
  - Administered: Applied or generally placed in area of ulceration or directly on top of closest superficial artery supplying affected tissues[25]
- Aspirin
  - Actions: Decreases platelet aggregation by inhibiting prostaglandin synthesis
  - Administered: Oral
  - Side effects: Gastrointestinal symptoms (eg, abdominal pain, nausea, constipation)

♦ Agents used in hyperlipidemia[54]
  • Niacin
    ▪ Actions: Decreases very low and low density lipoprotein levels
  • Reductase inhibitors
    ▪ Examples: Atorvastatin, pravastatin, simvastatin
    ▪ Actions: Decreases low density lipoproteins and triglycerides
  • Gemfibrozil
    ▪ Actions: Decreases very low density lipoproteins and lipase activity
♦ Blood glucose lowering agents: See Pattern D: Impaired Integumentary Integrity Associated With Full-Thickness Skin Involvement and Scar Formation
♦ Pharmacological agents to assist with smoking cessation
  • Transdermal nicotine patches to provide a gradual reduction in systemic nicotine exposure
  • Bupropion hydrochloride, a second-generation antidepressant, appears to reduce patient craving for nicotine
♦ Antimicrobial agents to control wound infection: See Pattern E: Impaired Integumentary Integrity Associated With Skin Involvement Extending Into Fascia, Muscle, or Bone and Scar Formation
♦ Pharmacological agents used to assist with pain management
  • NSAIDs
    ▪ Examples: Acetaminophen, aspirin, ibuprofen, naproxen
    ▪ Actions: Decrease inflammation, relieve mild to moderate pain, and may also decrease platelet aggregation
    ▪ Administered: Oral
    ▪ Side effects: Gastrointestinal symptoms, dizziness, headache, hematologic conditions
  • Narcotics
    ▪ Examples: Codeine, hydrocodone, oxycodone, oxymorphone, meperidine
    ▪ Actions: Used to relieve moderate to severe pain
    ▪ Administered: Oral or parenteral
    ▪ Side effects: Lightheadedness, gastrointestinal symptoms, sedation, respiratory depression

---

Case Study #1: Partial-Thickness Vascular Ulcer

Mr. Victor Giambi is a 45-year-old male, one-and-a-half pack per day smoker, who has a left lower extremity ulcer near his medial malleolus.

PHYSICAL THERAPIST EXAMINATION

HISTORY

♦ General demographics: Mr. Giambi is a 45-year-old white male whose primary language is English. He is right-hand dominant and has a high school diploma.
♦ Social history: He is divorced and lives alone.
♦ Employment/work: He works as a cashier at a local restaurant.
♦ Living environment: Mr. Giambi lives on the second floor of a three-story apartment building with elevator access and no stairs to enter.
♦ General health status
  • General health perception: Mr. Giambi reports that his health status is good.
  • Physical function: He reports that his physical function is normal for his age.
  • Psychological function: Normal.
  • Role function: Self-sufficient, cashier.
  • Social function: Mr. Giambi reports that he regularly goes over to friends' homes to play card games, and he enjoys watching sports.
♦ Social/health habits: He has smoked one-and-a-half packs per day for 25 years.
♦ Family history: His father died of a myocardial infarction (MI) at the age of 55.
♦ Medical/surgical history: Mr. Giambi had a carotid endartectomy 5 years ago and had a previous ulcer in the same location 4 years ago that took almost 1 year to close. He has no allergies.
♦ Current condition(s)/chief complaint(s): His ulcer occurred spontaneously about 5 months ago and has slowly increased in size. The previous treatment included covering the wound with an adhesive bandage two to four times per day. He complains of a mild ache in his left leg and of wound drainage that requires him to change his sock twice daily. He would like the wound to close.
♦ Functional status and activity level: Mr. Giambi is independent in all ADL and IADL, though he reports difficulty with changing his bandage and reaching his feet for donning socks. Although he played high school football and basketball, he has not exercised in the last 10 years.

- Medications: He takes one aspirin per day.
- Other clinical tests: Mr. Giambi reports he just completed his yearly physical, including a stress test and blood work that were normal.

SYSTEMS REVIEW

- Cardiopulmonary
  - BP: 135/78 mmHg
  - Edema: Noted in both LEs
  - HR: 76 bpm
  - RR: 12 bpm
- Integumentary
  - Presence of scar formation: Scarring is noted around current ulcer
  - Skin color: Brown staining consistent with hemosiderin deposition is noted at the distal 1/3 of both lower legs
  - Skin integrity: Open wound superior to the left medial malleolus
- Musculoskeletal
  - Gross range of motion: WNL
  - Gross strength: WNL
  - Gross symmetry: Symmetrical
  - Height: 5'10" (1.778 m)
  - Weight: 207 lbs (93.895 kg)
- Neuromuscular
  - Gross coordinated: WNL
  - Motor function: WNL
- Communication, affect, cognition, language, and learning style
  - Consciousness: Alert

- Orientation: Oriented x 3
- Learning preferences: Patient learns best by reading

TESTS AND MEASURES

- Anthropometric characteristics
  - BMI=30
  - Normal BMI ranges from 18.5 to 24.9. A BMI of 30 is defined as obese[55]
- Circulation
  - Pulse examination[3,23,34] (Table 3-4)
    - Performed as an indicator of arterial blood flow
    - Bilateral DP and PT pulses 1+
  - Capillary refill[1,17,35,56-59] (Table 3-5)
    - Performed as an indicator of superficial blood flow
    - Capillary refill was 2 seconds for both LEs
  - ABI[2,16,17,35,43,50,60-65] (Table 3-6)
    - Performed because pulses were diminished, suggesting arterial insufficiency
    - The ABI will help identify the presence of arterial insufficiency and assist with determining whether compression therapy is contraindicated
    - ABI=0.9
  - Trendelenburg test[51] (Table 3-7)
    - Performed to assess for venous insufficiency given hemosiderin deposition noted on Mr. Giambi's lower legs.
    - Venous distention occurred bilaterally after 15 seconds of standing suggesting deep or perforating vein incompetence
  - Homans' sign[33,66-68] (Table 3-8)

Table 3-4	
PULSE EXAMINATION	
Purpose	Indicator of arterial flow
Method	With the patient positioned comfortably supine, superficial arterial pulse is palpated
Interpretation	
Grade 0	Absent
	Nonpalpable
Grade 1+	Diminished pulse
	Palpable but intensity is decreased or may be easily obliterated with light pressure
Grade 2+	Normal pulse
	Pulse is easily palpable
Grade 3+	Bounding pulse
	Pulse is accentuated and very strong
Advantages	Quick, noninvasive, painless
Limitations	Pedal pulses may be difficult to palpate, especially if there is a significant amount of overlying soft tissue or edema. If this occurs, the clinician should try to obtain the pulse using a Doppler probe

Table 3-5	
CAPILLARY REFILL	
Purpose	Indicator of superficial blood flow
Method	Observe color of patient's skin in the area of interest
	Apply pressure with enough force to blanch the patient's skin
	Monitor the amount of time required before the patient's skin color returns to normal
Interpretation	<3 seconds=Normal capillary refill time
	>3 to 5 seconds=Surface tissue perfusion is impaired
Advantages	Quick, noninvasive, painless
	Reliable and valid assessment
Limitations	May be affected by tissue temperature and patient age

Table 3-6	
ANKLE-BRACHIAL INDEX	
Purpose	Indirect measure of peripheral tissue perfusion
Calculation	ABI=systolic pressure LE/systolic pressure UE
Method	Place BP cuff around the LE just proximal to the malleoli
	Apply ultrasound gel in the area of the PT artery
	Holding a Doppler probe at a 45-degree angle to the skin surface, move the probe until the swooshing sound of the pulse can be heard
	Inflate the cuff at least 20 mmHg above the point at which the swooshing sound is no longer audible
	Release the cuff and record the pressure at which the swooshing sound returns (systolic pressure of the PT artery)
	Repeat this procedure on both UEs to obtain the systolic pressure of the brachial artery at the cubital fossa; use the higher of these two values to calculate the ABI
Interpretation	
>1.1	Vessel calcification
0.9 to 1.1	Normal
0.7 to 0.9	Mild to moderate arterial insufficiency
0.5 to 0.7	Moderate arterial insufficiency
<0.5	Severe arterial insufficiency
Advantages	Quick, noninvasive
	Valid and reliable assessment
Limitations	Does not provide information about perfusion distal to the malleoli
	ABI >1.1 is not an adequate indicator of tissue perfusion
	ABI may be artificially elevated in patients with diabetes or arterial calcification

- Performed as a screening procedure to identify the presence of a DVT
- Negative bilaterally
- Alternative: Because of the potentially devastating consequences of a DVT (eg, pulmonary embolism) and the poor reliability of the Homans' sign, the reader is referred to the scoring system developed by Anand for an alternate screening strategy that more accurately predicts the presence of a DVT[68,69]

- Cranial and peripheral nerve integrity
  - Light touch: Intact
  - Thermal sensation: Normal
- Gait, locomotion, and balance: WNL
- Integumentary integrity
  - Associated skin
    - Skin color
      - Hemosiderin deposition noted at the distal 1/3 of both lower legs

- There is a 2-cm border of scarring evident around the wound bed
- Periwound maceration is evident extending 0.3 cm from the wound edge
  - Hair growth: Decreased on both lower legs
  - Nail growth: Normal
  - Temperature: WNL
  - Texture/turgor: WNL except scarred and hemosiderin stained areas are fragile and less pliable than the surrounding tissues
  - Edema
    - 1+ pitting edema bilateral lower legs and dorsal feet
    - Calf circumferential measurements symmetrical
- Activities, positioning, and postures that produce or relieve trauma to the skin: Occupation requires prolonged standing
- Wound
  - Open wound noted superior to the left medial malleolus

- Partial-thickness wound measures 3.8 x 5.2 cm, with a depth of 0.2 cm
- Wound bed contains approximately 95% granular tissue and 5% yellow slough tissue, primarily at the wound margins
- Signs of infection: None
- Muscle performance: Manual muscle testing results were normal
- Pain
  - Pain provocation tests: Mr. Giambi reports his pain increases with sitting during the history and decreases with elevation on the plinth during the examination
  - VAS[70-72]: Mr. Giambi rates his left lower leg pain as a 2/10 at rest
- Range of motion
  - Ankle dorsiflexion=R 0 to 15 degrees, L 0 to 12 degrees
  - Knee flexion=R 0 to 92 degrees, L 0 to 94 degrees limited by soft tissue opposition
  - Hip flexion=R 0 to 85 degrees, L 0 to 90 degrees limited by soft tissue opposition

Table 3-7
TRENDELENBURG TEST

Purpose	To assess for venous insufficiency
Method	Position the patient supine and elevate the LE to be assessed approximately 45 degrees. Note any superficial vein distention present
	Secure a tourniquet around the patient's distal thigh
	Have the patient stand for up to 1 minute; record the time when superficial venous distention occurs
	Release the tourniquet, and repeat the same procedure
Interpretation	Venous distention within 20 seconds of standing suggests deep or perforating vein incompetence
	Venous distention that occurs within 10 seconds of tourniquet removal suggests superficial vein incompetence
Advantages	Noninvasive, painless
Limitations	Reliability and validity unknown

Table 3-8
HOMANS' SIGN

Purpose	To identify the presence of a DVT
Method	Extend the patient's knee, then passively dorsiflex the ankle and palpate deep within the gastrocnemius muscle belly
Interpretation	The Homans' sign is positive if this technique produces or increases local calf pain
Advantages	Quick, noninvasive, painless
Limitations	Lacks sensitivity (33% to 96%) and specificity (20% to 72%)
	A positive Homans' sign may also be found in patients with superficial phlebitis and musculotendinous pathologies (eg, gastrocnemius strain)
	Refer to text for alternative DVT screening strategies

- Thoracolumbar flexion=0 to 60 degrees limited by soft tissue opposition
- Gastrocnemius length=R 0 to 8 degrees, L 0 to 7 degrees
♦ Self-care, home management/work, community, and leisure integration or reintegration
  - During the interview Mr. Giambi reports no difficulty with home care but states that he has difficulty reaching his wound to put on his bandage
  - He notes his work duties are inhibited by the need to change his bandage two to four times per shift secondary to drainage

EVALUATION

Mr. Giambi's history and risk factors previously outlined indicate that he is a sedentary, obese male smoker with a history of cardiovascular disease and prior ulceration. He has a partial-thickness wound due to venous insufficiency in addition to pitting edema and impaired LE and trunk ROM secondary to obesity. Mr. Giambi has difficulty with wound bandaging and is unable to work a normal shift secondary to the need for frequent bandage changes.

DIAGNOSIS

Mr. Giambi has a vascular ulcer that entails partial-thickness skin involvement and scar formation and has pain in his left lower leg. He has impaired: circulation; integumentary integrity; and range of motion. He is functionally limited in self-care and home management and in work, community, and leisure actions, tasks, and activities. These findings are consistent with placement in Pattern C: Impaired Integumentary Integrity Associated With Partial-Thickness Skin Involvement and Scar Formation. These impairments and functional limitations will be addressed in determining the prognosis and the plan of care.

PROGNOSIS AND PLAN OF CARE

Over the course of the visits, the following mutually established outcomes have been determined:
♦ Ability to perform physical activities related to self-care and work is improved
♦ Knowledge of behaviors that foster healthy habits, wellness, and prevention is increased
♦ Referrals are made to other professionals or resources
♦ Risk of recurrence is reduced
♦ Skin integrity is restored
♦ Tissue perfusion and oxygenation are enhanced

To achieve these outcomes, the appropriate interventions for this patient are determined. These will include: coordination, communication, and documentation; patient/client-related instruction; therapeutic exercise; functional training in self-care and home management; functional training in work, community, and leisure integration or reintegration; prescription, application, and, as appropriate, fabrication of devices and equipment; integumentary repair and protection techniques; and physical agents and mechanical modalities.

Based on the diagnosis and prognosis, Mr. Giambi is expected to require between five to eight visits over a 4-week period of time. Mr. Giambi lives alone, is motivated, and follows through with his home program. He is not severely impaired and is generally healthy.

INTERVENTIONS

RATIONALE FOR SELECTED INTERVENTIONS

Therapeutic Exercise

Exercise is extremely important for Mr. Giambi. Ankle plantar flexor contraction creates a hydrostatic force of approximately 200 mmHg within the veins propelling blood toward the heart. During relaxation, pressure is reduced to allow venous filling before the pressure is again exerted.[26]

Aerobic exercise[22] enhances the respiratory pump by increasing the rate and depth of respiration. Aerobic exercise involving the LEs increases the effect of the calf muscle pump. In addition, in combination with dietary modification, aerobic exercise will assist with weight loss.

Prescription, Application, and, as Appropriate, Fabrication of Devices and Equipment

Wound closure does not correct underlying wound etiology (venous HTN). Compression therapy decreases venous HTN by supporting the superficial veins, increasing venous return through enhancement of calf muscle pump effectiveness, and decreasing peripheral edema.[13] Mr. Giambi had a previous venous insufficiency ulcer, and the rate of recurrence without the use of ongoing compression to address venous HTN is 57% to 79%.[73] By utilizing compression therapy, the rate of recurrence may be as low as 28%.[73]

The compression needed at the ankle to counteract venous HTN is between 25 and 45 mmHg.[51] Patients with mild-moderate venous insufficiency without concomitant peripheral arterial disease[74] benefit from between 30 and 40 mmHg compression both to promote ulcer healing[75] and to prevent ulcer recurrence.[6,7,51,76,77]

Integumentary Repair and Protection Techniques

Debridement decreases wound bioburden, shortens the inflammatory phase of wound healing, decreases the energy required for wound healing, and eliminates the physical barrier to wound healing.[78-80] A moisturizer applied to Mr. Giambi's intact, hemosiderin stained skin will help to improve skin pliability and decrease the risk of future skin damage from minor trauma or irritation. A skin sealant applied to the periwound will help decrease maceration from wound drainage.

Moisture retentive dressings enhance wound healing in several ways. They maintain a moist, warm wound environment and facilitate autolytic debridement. They are associated with lower wound infection rates. Moisture retentive dressings absorb sufficient wound drainage to allow decreased dressing frequency and are associated with lower costs than traditional gauze bandages. They decrease patient pain complaint and do not traumatize the wound bed upon removal. Various wound dressings may be appropriate for his wound. The ideal dressing should cover the wound, maintain wound temperature and hydration, and allow dressing frequency chosen by the clinician. In addition, the dressing must be both available to the clinician/patient and be cost effective.[22,31,81-83]

Physical Agents and Mechanical Modalities

Pulsatile lavage with suction may be beneficial for Mr. Giambi for several reasons.[84-91] It removes loosely adhered debris, bacteria, exudate, and residual topical agents, and it softens eschar and facilitates debridement. The negative pressure may enhance granulation tissue formation, epithelialization, and local tissue perfusion. Pulsatile lavage may decrease pain associated with wound management techniques. Whirlpool is not indicated because the dependent positioning would exacerbate venous HTN and LE edema and the uncontrolled mechanical force from whirlpool agitation may traumatize the granular wound bed.

Compression may also be beneficial for Mr. Giambi for several reasons.[13,75,92] Compression therapy addresses wound etiology by supporting the superficial veins, enhancing calf muscle pump effectiveness, and decreasing peripheral edema. Short stretch compression bandages provide low resting pressures but high pressures during muscle activity, thus enhancing venous return. In addition, a multi-layer compression bandage system may be left in place for several days, an important consideration since he has difficulty reaching his wound for bandage changes.

COORDINATION, COMMUNICATION, AND DOCUMENTATION

Communication will occur with Mr. Giambi's primary care physician. He will be referred to his physician for assistance with a smoking cessation program that will be effective for him (eg, pharmacological, counseling, support group). He will be referred to a registered dietician to assist with weight management. All elements of the patient's management will be documented.

PATIENT/CLIENT-RELATED INSTRUCTION

Mr. Giambi will be instructed in the risk factors related to venous insufficiency, the importance of exercise, the need to eliminate smoking, and the appropriateness of diet modifications. Because his preferred learning style is review of written information, he will be provided with written copies of his instructional material, home exercise program (HEP), and self-care techniques. Particular emphasis will be placed upon the following as they relate to chronic venous insufficiency:

♦ Chronic venous insufficiency leads to venous HTN, edema, and impaired tissue oxygenation
♦ Compression therapy will improve venous return increasing wound healing potential in the short term and decreasing the risk of recurrence in the long term[76,78,93]
♦ Regular walking in combination with compression therapy will enhance venous return by way of increasing calf muscle pump efficiency and enhancing the respiratory pump
♦ Elevation of the LEs while sitting will enhance venous return[11]
♦ Prolonged static standing should be avoided as this increases venous HTN[11]
♦ He should be instructed to frequently weight shift, perform heel raises, walk in place, walk, or sit with his LEs elevated
♦ Smoking delays wound healing by causing vasoconstriction, increased platelet aggregation, and reduced oxygen availability[11,94]
♦ Open wounds or inappropriately bandaged wounds provide a direct pathway for bacteria to enter the body, increasing the risk of infection and sepsis
♦ Instruct him in the signs and symptoms of infection and action plan if these occur

Potential information related to weight management that may be given to Mr. Giambi includes the following[95]:
♦ Increase activity from sedentary level to increased caloric expenditure
♦ Decrease energy intake by eating low fat foods, decreasing snacks between meals, and using smaller portion sizes
♦ Water intake
  • 35 mL per kilogram of body weight/day[96]
  • Drink a glass of water before meals and with snacks to minimize food consumption and decrease the feeling of hunger that may occur with an empty stomach
♦ Minimize the use of alcohol to decrease non-nutritional caloric intake
♦ Increase fruit and vegetable intake to two to four and three to four servings per day, respectively

---

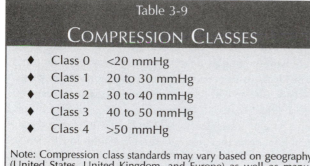

Table 3-9

COMPRESSION CLASSES

- ◆ Class 0   <20 mmHg
- ◆ Class 1   20 to 30 mmHg
- ◆ Class 2   30 to 40 mmHg
- ◆ Class 3   40 to 50 mmHg
- ◆ Class 4   >50 mmHg

Note: Compression class standards may vary based on geography (United States, United Kingdom, and Europe) as well as manufacturer. It is advisable to confirm the amount of compression in a given garment rather than rely on universal compression class guidelines.

THERAPEUTIC EXERCISE

- ◆ Aerobic capacity/endurance conditioning[55]
  - • Mode: Continuous
  - • Methods
    - ▪ Treadmill or over-land walking
    - ▪ Exercise bicycle
  - • Duration
    - ▪ Gradually increase time until able to walk or ride a minimum of 20 to 30 minutes
    - ▪ Progressively increase duration to 45 minutes once able to achieve desired exercise intensity
  - • Intensity
    - ▪ Goal is 60% to 80% of target HR
    - ▪ Target HR=[(maximum HR - resting HR) x % intensity] + resting HR
    - ▪ Patient is instructed in method to measure pulse and modulate exercise intensity based on HR response
  - • Frequency
    - ▪ 5 to 7 days per week
- ◆ Strength, power, and endurance training
  - • Ankle pumps, 20 times two to three times per day, preferably in combination with leg elevation
  - • Standing bilateral heel raises, 10 times, three times per day
- ◆ Mr. Giambi will maintain a log of therapeutic exercise to increase adherence to his home program and track progress over time

FUNCTIONAL TRAINING IN SELF-CARE AND HOME MANAGEMENT

- ◆ Self-care
  - • Before bathing, cover the bandage with plastic bags to keep it dry
- ◆ Home management
  - • Initiate an interrupted walking program, adding increasingly longer functional walks throughout the day, such as parking farther from home entrance or using the stairs rather than the elevator at home
  - • For convenient exercise at home
    - ▪ Consider buying an exercise bicycle or home treadmill
    - ▪ Consider buying an exercise video

FUNCTIONAL TRAINING IN WORK, COMMUNITY, AND LEISURE INTEGRATION OR REINTEGRATION

- ◆ Work
  - • Weight shift, march in place, or perform heel raises while standing at the cash register
  - • Park farther from the work entrance
  - • Take a short walk during one of his work breaks
  - • Bring a healthy lunch rather than buying fast food
- ◆ Leisure
  - • Prop LEs when sitting to enhance venous return
  - • Consider joining a fitness center

PRESCRIPTION, APPLICATION, AND, AS APPROPRIATE, FABRICATION OF DEVICES AND EQUIPMENT

- ◆ Fit Mr. Giambi for a below knee compression garment for the RLE prophylactically and the LLE upon wound closure
- ◆ He will be fitted for a class 2 (30 to 40 mmHg) below knee compression garment for the RLE (Table 3-9 describes the compression classes[97])
- ◆ Upon achieving wound closure, he will be fitted for a class 2 (30 to 40 mmHg) below knee compression garment for the LLE
- ◆ Mr. Giambi will be instructed in garment wear and care

INTEGUMENTARY REPAIR AND PROTECTION TECHNIQUES

- ◆ Debridement: Selective
  - • After pulsatile lavage treatment, the intact skin will be dried with a towel and any necessary sharp debridement should be performed
  - • Forceps or a scalpel will be used to assist with the removal of slough within the wound bed
- ◆ Dressings
  - • A hydrocolloid sheet will be applied to Mr. Giambi's wound
  - • The dressing will be signed, dated, and left in place for 5 to 7 days

- If strike-through occurs (wound drainage exceeds dressing capacity resulting in the soaking of moisture through the dressing to the external environment), the dressing will be changed more often[98,99]
  - ♦ Topical agents
    - Twice daily, a nonperfumed, low pH moisturizer will be applied to his lower legs and feet, except between his toes, on macerated skin, or on periwound skin
    - A skin sealant will be applied to the areas of maceration and periwound skin that will be covered with the primary dressing

PHYSICAL AGENTS AND MECHANICAL MODALITIES

- ♦ After removing his dressings, his leg will be positioned comfortably supine on a moisture-impermeable pad to absorb any irrigant runoff
- ♦ The physical therapist will wear appropriate personal protective equipment including, but not necessarily limited to, clean gloves, a face shield, hair covering, foot coverings, and a moisture-impermeable gown
- ♦ Physical agents: Hydrotherapy
  - The wound will be thoroughly irrigated using pulsatile lavage with an irrigation pressure of 4 to 15 psi
- ♦ Mechanical modalities: Compression bandaging
  - A multi-layer compression bandage system will be applied over his primary dressing
  - The dressing will be changed when the patient is seen in the physical therapy clinic every 5 to 7 days
  - If strike-through is present on the primary dressing, the patient will be seen more frequently

ANTICIPATED GOALS AND EXPECTED OUTCOMES

- ♦ Impact on pathology/pathophysiology
  - Debridement of nonviable tissue is achieved in four visits.
  - Edema is reduced to nonpitting in 2 weeks.
  - Pain is reduced to 0/10 in 4 weeks.
  - Periwound will be free of maceration in three visits.
  - Self-management of chronic venous insufficiency is improved.
  - Tissue perfusion and oxygenation are enhanced.
- ♦ Impact on impairments
  - Integumentary integrity is improved with wound closure within 4 weeks.
- ♦ Impact on functional limitations
  - Mr. Giambi is able to don and doff his compression garments with the use of a donning aide independently in eight visits.
- Mr. Giambi is able to work a full shift without needing to change his dressing in two visits.
- Tolerance to positions or activities is increased.
- ♦ Risk reduction/prevention
  - Risk of secondary impairment, including contralateral LE ulceration, is reduced.
  - Risk of ulcer recurrence is reduced.
- ♦ Impact on health, wellness, and fitness
  - Behaviors that foster healthy habits, wellness, and prevention are acquired.
  - Health status is improved.
  - Physical function is improved.
- ♦ Impact on societal resources
  - Referrals are made to other health care professionals or resources whenever necessary and appropriate.
  - Resources are utilized in a cost-effective way.
  - Utilization of physical therapy services is optimized.
- ♦ Patient/client satisfaction
  - Documentation occurs throughout patient management and follows APTA's *Guidelines for Physical Therapy Documentation.*[100]
  - Patient knowledge and awareness of the diagnosis, prognosis, interventions, and anticipated goals and outcomes are increased.
  - Patient understanding of anticipated goals and expected outcomes is increased.

REEXAMINATION

Reexamination is performed throughout the episode of care.

DISCHARGE

Mr. Giambi is discharged from physical therapy after a total of seven physical therapy sessions and attainment of his goals and expectations. These sessions have covered his entire episode of care. He is discharged because he has achieved his goals and expected outcomes.

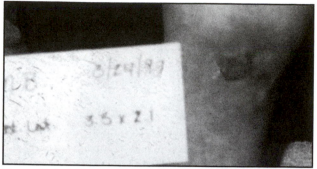

Figure 3-1. Mixed vascular disease and pressure ulcer. (See this figure in the Color Atlas following page 39.)

Case Study #2: Mixed Vascular Disease and Pressure Ulcer

Mrs. Marie Butcher is a 68-year-old female who has an ulcer on her left posterolateral calf (Figure 3-1).

PHYSICAL THERAPIST EXAMINATION

HISTORY

♦ General demographics: Mrs. Butcher is a 68-year-old female whose primary language is English. She is right-hand dominant and completed 2 years of college.

♦ Social history: She is married to a 72-year-old former Army medic and has three sons and six grandchildren who live in another state.

♦ Employment/work: She retired from a local manufacturing company 12 years ago due to a decline in her health.

♦ Living environment: She lives in a one-story house that is wheelchair accessible.

♦ General health status
  • General health perception: Mrs. Butcher reports that her health status is poor.
  • Physical function: She reports her physical function to be limited due to weakness, fatigue, and problems with BP control that she attributes to dialysis.
  • Role function: Wife, mother, grandmother.
  • Social function: Mrs. Butcher has been active in her local church where she assists with teaching an adult Sunday school class and with welcoming new members. She reports she has been unable to fully participate in these functions because of pain, and her feet swell if she sits more than 1 hour.

♦ Social/health habits: Mrs. Butcher is a nonsmoker and nondrinker.

♦ Family history: She reports both parents had "a little sugar" and died in their 60s.

♦ Medical/surgical history: Mrs. Butcher has Type 2 diabetes mellitus, retinopathy, neuropathy, nephropathy, and arteriosclerosis. She had a cardiac stent placement 2 years ago and a transient ischemic attack (TIA) 4 years ago. She has been undergoing dialysis three times per week for the past 2 years. She reports two falls in the past year that Mrs. Butcher relates to BP changes that occur after dialysis treatment. She is allergic to peanuts.

♦ Current condition(s)/chief complaint(s): Mrs. Butcher complains of a painful ulcer on the outside of her left leg that began insidiously about 2 months ago. The wound has slowly increased in size. She reports the ulcer is extremely painful and makes sitting on the dialysis reclining chair for 2 hours difficult. Current wound treatment consists of Mr. Butcher rinsing the wound with hydrogen peroxide and covering it with a gauze wrap daily. She would like the wound to close and the pain to decrease.

♦ Functional status and activity level: Mrs. Butcher reports limitations in ADL and IADL. She does not participate in an exercise program.

♦ Medications: Insulin, metformin, cyclothiazide, propranolol, warfarin, Neurontin.

♦ Other clinical tests: Due to pain and a history of two falls, an x-ray was performed of her left leg that was negative for bony changes. Her calcified tibial artery can be seen on the radiograph. The following laboratory test results are available from the patient's medical record (see Table 3-10 for normal values):
  • Hct=32%

Table 3-10	
LABORATORY REFERENCE VALUES	
Hematocrit	Women: 35% to 47%
	Men: 42% to 52%
Hemoglobin	Women: 12 to 15 g/dL
	Men: 14 to 16.5 g/dL
White blood cell count	4500 to 11,000/mm³
Total lymphoctye count	>1800
Serum albumin	3.5 to 5.5 mg/dL
Serum prealbumin	15 to 43 mg/dL
Serum transferrin	>170 mg/dL
Fasting blood glucose	70 to 110 mg/dL
Urine glucose	Negative
Blood urea nitrogen	8.0 to 25.0 mg/dL
Creatinine	0.6 to 1.2 mg/dL

Table 3-11
DOPPLER ULTRASOUND

Purpose	
Arterial Doppler	To identify faint or nonpalpable peripheral pulses to assess arterial patency
Venous Doppler	To identify obstruction of venous blood flow or valve incompetence
Method (Arterial)	Apply ultrasound gel to the area where the artery in question would normally be palpated
	Hold the probe at a 45 degree angle to the skin surface
	Slowly move the probe until the swooshing sound of the pulse can be heard
Interpretation	A swooshing sound indicates the arterial pulse. The pulse should be documented as being present with the use of a Doppler probe
	The lack of an audible signal indicates no movement of fluid within the artery, and hence, no perfusion. The peripheral arterial pulse should be documented as being absent with Doppler ultrasound
Advantages	Quick, inexpensive, noninvasive clinical test of vascular flow
Limitations	Venous Doppler testing is more subjective and the results less reliable than with an arterial Doppler exam

- Hgb=11.2 g/dL
- WBC=8000/mm^3
- Fasting glucose=200 mg/dL
- Urine glucose=Negative
- BUN=98 mg/dL
- Creatinine=7.0 mg/dL

SYSTEMS REVIEW

- ◆ Cardiovascular/pulmonary
  - BP: 150/58 mmHg
  - Edema: Present BLE
  - HR: 80 bpm
  - RR: 15 bpm
- ◆ Integumentary
  - Presence of scar formation: Scarring noted around ulcer
  - Skin color: There is a slight amount of hemosiderin deposition noted on the left calf, posterior greater than anterior
  - Skin integrity: Irregular-shaped open wound posterolateral left lower leg
- ◆ Musculoskeletal
  - Gross range of motion: WNL except limited ankle dorsiflexion
  - Gross strength: LE and UE grossly 4/5, fatigues with testing
  - Gross symmetry: Symmetrical
  - Height: 5'0" (1.524 m)
  - Weight: 112 lbs (50.803 kg)
- ◆ Neuromuscular
  - Transfers from wheelchair with difficulty

- Gait is unsteady with cane
- ◆ Communication, affect, cognition, language, and learning style
  - Communication, affect, cognition: WNL
  - Learning preferences: Patient learns best by listening, husband by demonstration

TESTS AND MEASURES

- ◆ Anthropometric characteristics
  - BMI=22
  - Normal BMI ranges from 18.5 to 24.9[55]
- ◆ Assistive and adaptive devices
  - Cane and wheelchair for distances
- ◆ Circulation
  - Pulse exam[3,23,34] (see Table 3-4)
    - Performed as an indicator of arterial blood flow
    - Popliteal bilaterally=1+, DP bilaterally=1+, PT R=1+ and L=0
  - Doppler ultrasound[41,63] (Table 3-11)
    - Performed on the left PT artery because the pulse was nonpalpable
    - Left PT artery pulse identifiable with Doppler
  - Capillary refill[1,17,35,56-59] (see Table 3-5)
    - Performed as an indicator of superficial blood flow
    - Capillary refill was 5 seconds bilateral LEs
  - ABI[2,16,17,35,43,50,60-65] (see Table 3-6)
    - Performed due to history of vascular disease, calcification of the tibial artery is visible on radiograph, and because pulses were found to be diminished

- The ABI will help determine the severity of arterial insufficiency and assist with determining the plan of care
  - ABI=1.2 LLE
- Trendelenburg test: Unable to perform secondary to pain with tourniquet application
- Homans' sign[33,66-68]
  - Performed as a screening procedure on patients with suspected peripheral vascular to identify the presence of a DVT because of the potentially devastating consequences of a DVT (eg, pulmonary embolism)
  - Negative bilaterally
  - Alternative: Because of the potentially devastating consequences of a DVT (eg, pulmonary embolism) and the poor reliability of the Homans' sign, the reader is referred to the scoring system developed by Anand for an alternate screening strategy that more accurately predicts the presence of a DVT[68,69]
- Rubor of dependency[17,34] (Table 3-12)
  - Performed secondary to history of vascular disease, diminished pulses, and invalid ABI
  - Pain and pallor of the foot found after 28 seconds of elevation with rubor shortly after dependent positioning
- Venous filling time[17] (Table 3-13)
  - Performed because ABI findings were invalid as an indicator of arterial insufficiency
  - Venous filling time was 25 seconds on the R, 29 seconds on the L

- Cranial and peripheral nerve integrity
  - Light touch
    - Performed due to her history of diabetes
    - Able to identify 5.07 Semmes-Weinstein monofilament BLE (see Table 4-5)
  - Thermal sensation: Normal
- Gait, locomotion, and balance
  - Transfers with difficulty requiring use of BUE
  - Ambulates with cane 25 feet with contact guard assist, increased left-right sway, decreased step-lengths, and decreased speed
  - Performance-Oriented Mobility Assessment[101-104]
    - Since Mrs. Butcher has an unsteady gait, the test was performed to better quantify her gait deviations and to assess for fall risk
    - Gait score=5/12 indicating an abnormal gait and impaired mobility
  - Berg Balance test[105,106]
    - Since Mrs. Butcher has an unsteady gait, test was performed to determine fall risk and target areas for balance training
    - Score=42/56
    - A score of less than 45 on the Berg Balance test is predictive of recurrent falls
- Integumentary integrity
  - Associated skin
    - Skin color
      - Slight amount of hemosiderin deposition noted on the left calf, posterior greater than anterior, scarring noted around ulcer
    - Hair growth: Absent both LEs

Table 3-12	
RUBOR OF DEPENDENCY	
Purpose	Indirect assessment of arterial blood flow in the LE
Method	Position the patient supine and note the color of the plantar aspect of the patient's foot
	Elevate the LE approximately 60 degrees for 1 minute
	Note the color of the plantar surface of the patient's foot
	Return the LE to the test surface; if a color change occurred with elevation, note the time required for the skin to return to its pre-test color
Interpretation	
Normal	Minimal or no color change with testing
Mild AI	Pallor after 45 seconds of elevation
Moderate AI	Pallor within 30 to 45 seconds of elevation
Severe AI	Pallor within 25 seconds of elevation and the plantar surface of the foot will become bright red shortly after being returned to the supine position
Advantages	Quick, noninvasive, painless
Limitations	Test reliability and validity unknown
AI=arterial insufficiency	

Table 3-13	
VENOUS FILLING TIME	
Purpose	Predictor of AI and as an indicator of VI
Method	Position the patient in supine and note the superficial veins on the dorsal surface of the patient's foot
	Elevate the limb approximately 60 degrees for 1 minute, or until the veins have been drained by gravity
	Next, place the patient's extremity in the dependent position and record the time required for the superficial veins to refill
Interpretation	
Normal	5 to 15 seconds
VI	<5 seconds
AI	>20 seconds
Advantages	Quick, noninvasive, painless
	Particularly useful in patients who have an ABI of >1.1
Limitations	Test reliability and validity unknown

AI=arterial insufficiency, VI=venous insufficiency,

- Nail growth: Normal
- Temperature: Toes are cool to palpation
- Texture/turgor: Skin appears thin and fragile, mildly anhydrous
- Edema
  - 1+ pitting edema dorsal feet
  - Calf circumferential measurements symmetrical
- Risk assessment scales
  - Performed due to her impaired mobility and multiple medical conditions
  - Braden Scale for Predicting Pressure Sore Risk=19
    - The Braden scale is a valid and reliable tool for the assessment of the risk of pressure ulcers
    - Scores range from 6 to 23 with lower scores indicating greater risk of pressure ulcer development
    - Patients with scores less than 18 are generally considered at greater risk for pressure ulcers
- Activities, positioning, and postures that produce or relieve trauma to the skin
  - Mrs. Butcher reports that for dialysis she generally lies on the reclining dialysis chair with her legs crossed at the ankle with her left leg on top of her right but has been unable to do so for the past 2 weeks due to pain
- Wound
  - Irregular-shaped, open wound noted left posterolateral lower leg
  - Partial-thickness wound measures 3.5 x 2.1 cm,

with a depth of 0.2 cm
  - Wound bed contains 100% granular tissue
  - Signs of infection: None
- Muscle performance
  - Manual muscle testing revealed the following impairments
    - B shoulder flexion, abduction, extension; elbow flexion; hip flexion; hip abduction=4-/5
    - B knee flexion, knee extension, dorsiflexion, nonweightbearing plantarflexion, inversion, eversion, and great toe extension=4/5
  - Patient fatigued with testing
- Pain
  - Pain provocation tests
    - Mrs. Butcher reports pain at the wound site and in both lower legs
    - The pain increases with lying on the dialysis chair, when her legs are propped on the bed or a foot stool, with sitting more than 1 hour, and with walking
  - VAS[70-72]: Mrs. Butcher rates her pain as a 6/10 at rest, and 8/10 with ambulation and wound management procedures
- Range of motion
  - Ankle dorsiflexion=R 0 to 0 degrees, L 0 to 5 degrees
  - Gastrocnemius length=R lacks 2 degrees from neutral, L 0 to 2 degrees
- Self-care and home management
  - Self-care
    - During the interview Mrs. Butcher reports that

she requires her husband's assistance for donning shoes and socks, bed mobility, bathing, and wound care
  - Home management
    - She is unable to perform even light housework or grocery shopping secondary to feelings of fatigue, weakness, and instability
    - Mrs. Butcher uses a cane to ambulate in her home
- Work, community, and leisure integration or reintegration
  - Community
    - Her husband pushes her in a wheelchair for mobility outside of the home and at church

EVALUATION

Mrs. Butcher's history and risk factors previously outlined indicate that she is a sedentary female with cardiovascular, peripheral vascular, eye, and kidney disease. She has a nonhealing, partial-thickness wound due to the combined effects of mixed vascular disease and pressure from prolonged positioning of the left posterolateral calf on the right tibial crest during dialysis. She has decreased ankle ROM, global impairments in muscle performance, and limitations in self-care. She has decreased balance and is at risk for falls. She has decreased mobility and is at risk for the development of pressure ulcers.[107,108]

DIAGNOSIS

Mrs. Butcher has a mixed vascular disease and pressure ulcer associated with partial-thickness skin involvement and scar formation and has pain at the wound site and in both LEs. She has impaired: circulation; gait, locomotion, and balance; integumentary integrity; muscle performance; and range of motion. She is functionally limited in self-care and home management and in work, community, and leisure actions, tasks, and activities. These findings are consistent with placement in Pattern C: Impaired Integumentary Integrity Associated With Partial-Thickness Skin Involvement and Scar Formation. These impairments and functional limitations will be addressed in determining the prognosis and the plan of care.

PROGNOSIS AND PLAN OF CARE

Over the course of the visits, the following mutually established outcomes have been determined:
- Gait, locomotion, and balance are improved
- Knowledge of behaviors that foster healthy habits, wellness, and prevention is increased
- Patient/family knowledge and awareness of diagnosis, prognosis, interventions, and anticipated goals and outcomes are increased
- Physical function is improved
- Risk factors are reduced
- Risk of secondary impairment is reduced
- ROM is improved
- Skin integrity is restored
- Tissue perfusion and oxygenation are enhanced

To achieve these outcomes, the appropriate interventions for this patient are determined. These will include: coordination, communication, and documentation; patient/client-related instruction; therapeutic exercise; functional training in self-care and home management; functional training in work, community, and leisure integration or reintegration; integumentary repair and protection techniques; and physical agents and mechanical modalities.

Based on the diagnosis and prognosis, Mrs. Butcher is expected to require between four to six visits over a 4-week period of time. Mrs. Butcher is moderately impaired and has multiple co-morbidities. However, she has excellent social support, lives with her husband, is motivated, and follows through with her home program.

INTERVENTIONS

RATIONALE FOR SELECTED INTERVENTIONS

Therapeutic Exercise

Exercise is extremely important for Mrs. Butcher. Suboptimal ankle dorsiflexion ROM impairs the calf muscle pump.[7,26] Ankle plantar flexor contraction creates a hydrostatic force of approximately 200 mmHg within the veins propelling blood toward the heart. During relaxation, pressure is reduced to allow venous filling before the pressure is again exerted.[26]

Gains in flexibility may be maximized by performing three stretches of 30-second duration.[109] In addition, walking increases the effect of the calf muscle pump.[26]

Integumentary Repair and Protection Techniques

A moisturizer applied to Mrs. Butcher's intact skin will help improve skin pliability and decrease the risk of future skin damage from minor trauma or irritation. A skin sealant will help decrease maceration from wound drainage. Macerated skin is more fragile and friable than healthy skin.

Wound irrigation with normal saline is a treatment of choice for this patient since it removes loosely adhered debris, bacteria, dressing residue, and old topical agents.

Irrigation may decrease the risk of infection and promote moist wound healing. It is preferred over whirlpool for Mrs. Butcher as it does not increase peripheral edema, and the irrigation pressure is more controlled so as not to traumatize the fragile granulation tissue within the wound bed. Gentle irrigation is preferred over pulsatile lavage with suction because she complains of 6/10 resting wound pain and 8/10 with dressing changes. In addition, gentle irrigation is less expensive than pulsatile lavage with suction.[86,89,90,110,111]

Moisture-retentive dressings enhance wound healing in several ways. They maintain a moist, warm wound environment and are associated with lower rates of wound infection. They absorb sufficient wound drainage to allow decreased dressing frequency and are associated with lower costs than traditional gauze bandages. Moisture-retentive dressings decrease patient pain complaint and do not traumatize the wound bed upon removal. They are easier to apply and will not obstruct blood flow like a gauze wrap may.[22,31,81,82,112-114]

Specifically, a semipermeable foam for this patient has advantages that will enhance wound healing. It provides thermal insulation and cushioning to decrease the adverse effects of pressure when Mrs. Butcher is lying down. Unlike a hydrocolloid, a semipermeable foam is minimally adhesive and, therefore, will not traumatize fragile skin upon removal. Unlike a gauze wrap, a semipermeable foam is not secured circumferentially around her limb and, therefore, will not constrict blood flow with changes in her edema that may occur with dialysis and venous insufficiency.[22,81,112-114]

The hydrogen peroxide rinse will be discontinued because of the cytotoxic effects antiseptics have on open wounds.[115]

COORDINATION, COMMUNICATION, AND DOCUMENTATION

Mrs. Butcher's husband will be encouraged to be actively involved in all aspects of her care. Her primary care physician will be contacted regarding her pain complaint to request an alteration in pharmacological interventions if appropriate. All elements of the patient's management will be documented.

PATIENT/CLIENT-RELATED INSTRUCTION

Mrs. and Mr. Butcher will be instructed in the risk factors for pressure and vascular insufficiency ulcers. Particular emphasis will be placed on:

♦ Instruction in proper bandaging since open wounds or poorly bandaged wounds provide a direct pathway for bacteria to enter the body, increasing the risk of infection and sepsis
♦ Instructing patient and her husband in the signs and symptoms of infection and action plan if these occur
♦ Instructing patient and her husband in proper wound management

♦ Since arterial and venous insufficiency limit blood flow, proper nutrition, and oxygenation to affected areas, instructing the patient in ways to optimize her blood flow by:
  ● Avoiding constrictive clothing, such as tight elastic socks or elastic pant leg cuffs
  ● Avoiding leg elevation
♦ Since prolonged or excessive pressure obstructs blood flow causing local tissue ischemia, instructing the patient in ways to decrease the risk of skin damage due to pressure by[110]:
  ● Frequent position changes
  ● Minimizing pressure over bony prominences
  ● Using pressure-reducing devices
♦ Avoiding skin trauma by:
  ● Protecting against excessive heat or cold (bath water, heating pads, and the environment)
  ● Being aware of potential obstacles, such as wheelchair leg rests and table edges that if bumped against may traumatize fragile skin
  ● Not using chemicals, such as corn removers, unless directed to do so by a clinician
  ● Having her husband inspect her skin daily for signs of trauma, irritation, or excessive pressure
  ● Lifting body weight rather than dragging skin along support surfaces
♦ Knowing the importance of proper nutrition for wound healing and decreasing the progression of complications due to diabetes

THERAPEUTIC EXERCISE

♦ Flexibility exercises
  ● Ankle pumps 20 times per waking hour
  ● Stretching exercises should be done after warming up, using a slow and steady stretch accompanied by deep breathing, and building hold up to 30 seconds
  ● Dorsiflexion stretches
    ■ Method: Sitting in a chair, extend knee, use a bathrobe tie looped around the ball of the foot to assist with ankle dorsiflexion
    ■ Parameters
      ▸ 30-second hold
      ▸ Three repetitions
      ▸ Both legs
      ▸ Once daily
♦ Gait and locomotion training
  ● Walk with cane and husband's assistance 25 feet
  ● Two to three times per day
  ● If able, progress distance
  ● If feeling dizzy or unwell, limit ambulation for that day

FUNCTIONAL TRAINING IN SELF-CARE AND HOME MANAGEMENT

- ◆ Self-care and home management
  - Her husband will be shown how to perform daily skin checks on Mrs. Butcher to identify early signs of the adverse effects of pressure or trauma
  - Sleeping or lying on the left side or with the left hip externally rotated should be avoided as this causes pressure on the left posterolateral lower leg and open wound
  - Mr. Butcher will be shown how to assist his wife with bed mobility while minimizing skin friction and shear forces
  - While in dialysis, position LLE so as to avoid pressure on the wound
  - Mrs. Butcher should shift positions often when awake
  - When sitting for more than 30 minutes, she should perform ankle pumps to decrease LE edema and improve venous return
  - Mobility training
    - Because of her fluctuating BP response to dialysis and her significant multi-system disease, it was predicted that she would not be able to consistently ambulate independently even with gait and balance training
    - Therefore, Mr. Butcher will be instructed in the use of contact guard assistance to ensure Mrs. Butcher is safe when ambulating
    - Intermittent, short, assisted walks will be encouraged

FUNCTIONAL TRAINING IN WORK, COMMUNITY, AND LEISURE INTEGRATION OR REINTEGRATION

- ◆ Leisure
  - Mrs. Butcher will be encouraged to ambulate with her husband's assistance and her cane within her church school classroom and within the sanctuary as able

INTEGUMENTARY REPAIR AND PROTECTION TECHNIQUES

- ◆ Dressings
  - A semipermeable foam will be applied to Mrs. Butcher's wound
  - The dressing will be signed, dated, and left in place for 5 days
  - If strike-through occurs, the dressing will be changed more often
  - After the second visit, if the wound is showing signs of improvement, her husband will be instructed in home dressing changes and treatment frequency for wound management may be reduced
  - Because Mr. Butcher learns best by demonstration, the clinician will have him observe Mrs. Butcher's dressing procedure first before having him perform a repeat demonstration to ensure proper technique
  - Pictures of the dressing change procedure may be beneficial
- ◆ Topical agents
  - Twice daily, a nonperfumed, low pH moisturizer will be applied to her lower legs and feet, except between her toes and on periwound skin
  - A skin sealant will be applied to the areas of periwound skin that will be covered with the primary dressing

PHYSICAL AGENTS AND MECHANICAL MODALITIES

- ◆ Hydrotherapy
  - The wound will be irrigated with normal saline using a 35-mL syringe with a 19-gauge angiocatheter

ANTICIPATED GOALS AND EXPECTED OUTCOMES

- ◆ Impact on pathology/pathophysiology
  - Pain is reduced to 5/10 in 4 weeks.
  - Tissue perfusion and oxygenation are enhanced.
- ◆ Impact on impairments
  - Gastrocnemius length is improved to 0 to 8 degrees bilaterally in 2 weeks.
  - Integumentary integrity is improved with wound area decreased by 75% within 4 weeks.
- ◆ Impact on functional limitations
  - Mrs. Butcher is able to walk 50 feet with a cane and Mr. Butcher's contact guard assistance in 3 weeks.
  - Tolerance to positions or activities is increased.
- ◆ Risk reduction/prevention
  - Mr. and Mrs. Butcher are independent with bed mobility and transfers while minimizing friction and shear forces to Mrs. Butcher's skin in two visits.
  - Mr. and Mrs. Butcher are independent with skin checks in two visits.
  - Risk of ulcer recurrence is reduced.
  - Safety is improved.
  - Self-management of peripheral vascular disease is improved.
- ◆ Impact on health, wellness, and fitness
  - Behaviors that foster healthy habits, wellness, and prevention are acquired.

- Health status is improved.
- Patient/caregiver management of ulcer is improved.
- Physical function is improved.
♦ Impact on societal resources
- Utilization of physical therapy services is optimized.
- Referrals are made to other health care professionals or resources whenever necessary and appropriate.
- Resources are utilized in a cost-effective way.
♦ Patient/client satisfaction
- Documentation occurs throughout patient management and follows APTA's *Guidelines for Physical Therapy Documentation.*[100]
- Patient and caregiver knowledge and awareness of the diagnosis, prognosis, interventions, and anticipated goals and outcomes are increased.
- Patient understanding of anticipated goals and expected outcomes is increased.

REEXAMINATION

Reexamination is performed throughout the episode of care.

DISCHARGE

Mrs. Butcher is discharged from physical therapy after a total of four physical therapy sessions and attainment of her goals and expectations. These sessions have covered her entire episode of care. She is discharged because she has achieved her goals and expected outcomes.

PSYCHOLOGICAL ASPECTS

To maximize compliance and outcomes, her husband will be involved in all aspects of her care.

Case Study #3:
Superficial Partial-Thickness Burn Wound

Ms. Lainna Malloy is a 42-year-old female who has a burn on the dorsum of her right hand (Figure 3-2).

PHYSICAL THERAPIST EXAMINATION

HISTORY

♦ General demographics: Ms. Malloy is a 42-year-old female whose primary language is English. She is a right-hand dominant college graduate.

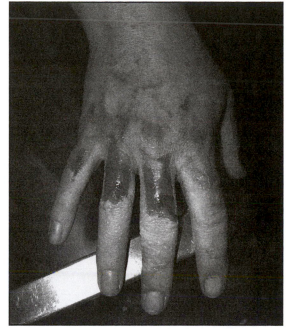

Figure 3-2. Superficial partial-thickness burn wound. (See this figure in the Color Atlas following page 39.)

♦ Social history: Ms. Malloy is a divorced mother of two: a 15-year-old son living at home and an 18-year-old daughter living at college.
♦ Employment/work: She is a self-employed painter.
♦ Living environment: Ms. Malloy lives in a two-story house with 12 steps and a rail to access the second floor. There are three steps and no rail to enter her home.
♦ General health status
- General health perception: She reports that her health status is good.
- Physical function: She reports difficulty with the use of her right hand since her injury.
- Psychological function: Normal.
- Role function: Mother, painter.
- Social function: She is active in the local parent-teacher association. She enjoys reading and drawing.
♦ Social/health habits: She is a nonsmoker and nondrinker.
♦ Family history: Unremarkable.
♦ Medical/surgical history: She had a hysterectomy at the age of 40. She has no allergies.
♦ Current condition(s)/chief complaint(s): Ms. Malloy reports that she spilled a pot of hot water 5 days ago sustaining a right hand burn. She went to the emergency room and was bandaged with 1% silver sulfadiazine, and her hand was wrapped in a gauze dressing. Two times per day, she has been rinsing her hand with water, applying a thick coat of silver sulfadiazine, and wrap-

ping her hand in a gauze dressing. She would like the wound to close so that she can return to her previous functional activities.

♦ Functional status and activity level: Ms. Malloys reports current limitations in ADL, IADL, and painting due to limitations in the use of her right hand. She has been afraid to shower since the injury for fear of wound infection. Normally, she jogs and weight trains 3 days per week, but has not been able to weight train due to her burn.

♦ Medications: Multivitamin with iron.

♦ Other clinical tests: None.

SYSTEMS REVIEW

♦ Cardiovascular/pulmonary
  • BP: 128/75 mmHg
  • Edema: Slight, right digits
  • HR: 72 bpm
  • RR: 12 bpm
♦ Integumentary
  • Presence of scar formation: None
  • Skin color: WNL
  • Skin integrity: Open wounds right hand, dorsal third, fourth, and fifth digits
  • Skin texture: Maceration noted dorsal right second digit and all periwound tissue
♦ Musculoskeletal
  • Gross range of motion: Limited right digits 2 to 5 flexion
  • Gross strength: WNL
  • Gross symmetry: Symmetrical
  • Height: 5'6" (1.676 m)
  • Weight: 143 lbs (64.865 kg)
♦ Neuromuscular
  • Balance, gait, locomotion: Not impaired
  • Transfers, transitions: Not impaired
♦ Communication, affect, cognition, language, and learning style
  • Communication, affect, cognition: WNL
  • Learning preferences: Ms. Malloy learns best by reading

TESTS AND MEASURES

♦ Anthropometric characteristics
  • BMI=23
  • Normal BMI ranges from 18.5 to 24.9[55]
♦ Circulation
  • Pulse exam[3,23,34] (see Table 3-4)
    ■ Performed as an indicator of arterial blood flow
    ■ Radial and ulnar pulses 2+ bilaterally

• Capillary refill[1,17,35,56-59] (see Table 3-5)
  ■ Performed as an indicator of superficial blood flow and to assist with determining wound depth
  ■ Wounds 1 second; fingertips 3 seconds bilaterally
♦ Cranial and peripheral nerve integrity
  • Light touch: Intact
  • Thermal sensation: Normal
♦ Integumentary integrity
  • Associated skin
    ■ Skin color: Slight increase in pigmentation dorsal metacarpophalangeal (MCP) joints 3 to 5
    ■ Hair growth: Intact hair follicles within wound beds
    ■ Nail growth: Normal
    ■ Temperature: Normal
    ■ Texture/turgor: Maceration noted dorsal right second digit and all periwound tissue
    ■ Edema: Circumferential measurements midshaft proximal phalanx
      ▸ Digit 1=R 5.7 cm, L 5.7 cm
      ▸ Digit 2=R 5.8 cm, L 5.8 cm
      ▸ Digit 3=R 6.1 cm, L 5.8 cm
      ▸ Digit 4=R 5.9 cm, L 5.7 cm
      ▸ Digit 5=R 4.7 cm, L 4.7 cm
  • Wound
    ■ Because of the limited surface area involved in her burns,[116] wound size was determined using length x width measurements
    ■ Partial-thickness wounds measure
      ▸ Dorsal third digit=3.0 cm x 1.4 cm
      ▸ Dorsal fourth digit=4.0 cm x 1.2 cm
      ▸ Dorsal fifth digit=1.0 cm x 0.6 cm
    ■ Wound depth: Superficial partial-thickness[117-119]
    ■ Wound characteristics
      ▸ Wound bed is void of nonviable tissue or slough
      ▸ Signs of infection: None
      ▸ There is minimal bleeding of the wound on the third digit
♦ Muscle performance
  • Grip strength with a dynamometer: R=28 kg with pain complaint, L=42 kg
  • Normal manual muscle testing bilaterally
♦ Pain
  • She rates her right hand pain as a 3/10 on a VAS[70-72]
♦ Range of motion: Bilateral hands unimpaired except the following:

- R MCP flexion
  - Digit 3=0 to 80 degrees
  - Digit 4=0 to 78 degrees
- R proximal interphalangeal (PIP) joint flexion digit 4=0 to 90 degrees
♦ Self-care and home management
  - During the interview Ms. Malloy reports difficulty with all ADL and IADL involving the right hand
  - Specifically, she reports inability to eat or brush her teeth with her right hand, difficulty writing, and inability to perform fine motor tasks, such as drawing or painting, due to dressing bulk and discomfort
  - She has difficulty bandaging her wound with her nondominant left hand
    - Therefore, she has been wrapping her third, fourth, and fifth digits together in a bulky gauze wrap

EVALUATION

Ms. Malloy's history and risk factors previously outlined indicate that she is a healthy female. Ms. Malloy has a superficial partial-thickness burn on her right hand. She has decreased right MCP and PIP ROM and right grip strength. She has limitations in self-care, work, and leisure activities that require the use of the right hand.

DIAGNOSIS

Ms. Malloy has a superficial partial-thickness burn with scar formation on her right hand and has pain in her right hand. She has impaired: integumentary integrity; muscle performance; and range of motion. She is functionally limited in self-care and home management and in work, community, and leisure actions, tasks, and activities. These findings are consistent with placement in Pattern C: Impaired Integumentary Integrity Associated With Partial-Thickness Skin Involvement and Scar Formation. These impairments and functional limitations will be addressed in determining the prognosis and the plan of care.

PROGNOSIS AND PLAN OF CARE

Over the course of the visits, the following mutually established outcomes have been determined:
♦ Patient/family knowledge and awareness of diagnosis, prognosis, interventions, and anticipated goals and outcomes are increased
♦ Physical function is improved
♦ Risk factors are reduced
♦ Risk of secondary impairment is reduced

♦ ROM is improved
♦ Skin integrity is restored
♦ Tissue perfusion and oxygenation are enhanced

To achieve these outcomes, the appropriate interventions for this patient are determined. These will include: coordination, communication, and documentation; patient/client-related instruction; therapeutic exercise; functional training in self-care and home management; functional training in work, community, and leisure integration or reintegration; integumentary repair and protection techniques; and physical agents and mechanical modalities.

Based on the diagnosis and prognosis, Ms. Malloy is expected to require between two to five visits over a 2-week period of time. Ms. Malloy lives with her teenage son, is motivated, and follows through with her home program. She is not severely impaired and is generally healthy.

INTERVENTIONS

RATIONALE FOR SELECTED INTERVENTIONS

Therapeutic Exercise

Exercise is extremely important for Ms. Malloy. ROM exercises will increase active range of motion (AROM), decrease wound contraction, improve skin extensibility, and improve functional use of the affected area.[120,121]

Integumentary Repair and Protection Techniques

Sterile technique is not warranted for this patient given the wound size, depth, and her lack of any significant medical conditions that might inhibit normal, acute wound healing.[116]

Debridement will be used since it decreases wound bioburden, shortens the inflammatory phase of wound healing, decreases the energy required for wound healing, and eliminates the physical barrier to wound healing.[78-80,121]

Saline irrigation after whirlpool has been shown to remove four times as much bacteria as whirlpool alone.[122]

A skin sealant will help decrease maceration from wound drainage and the topical antimicrobial. Macerated skin is more fragile and friable than healthy skin. A moisturizer applied to her intact skin will help improve skin pliability, decrease scarring, and decrease the risk of future skin damage from minor trauma or irritation.[22]

After communication with her referring physician, the silver sulfadiazine will be replaced with bacitracin.[123,124] Bacitracin, like silver sulfadiazine, is a broad spectrum antimicrobial. It can be changed as little as one time per day and still retain its antimicrobial effects, while silver sulfadiazine requires twice daily bandage changes. Bacitracin is a thin ointment that will maintain wound hydration but will decrease the potential for periwound maceration that has occurred with the use of the thick cream, silver sulfadiazine.

Petrolatum-impregnated gauze will be used, since it will decrease wound bed trauma with dressing changes, ROM, and functional use of the right hand.[112,125] If a cotton swab is used to apply a topical agent, wisps of cotton may remain within the wound bed causing the body to mount an inflammatory response.[126,127] By using a sterile calcium alginate swab (or sterile tongue blade) to apply the bacitracin, this undesired inflammatory response can be prevented.

A thin gauze dressing is the dressing of choice for this patient, since it will enhance fine motor tasks, allow increased functional use of the hand, and allow coverage of the irregular-shaped wounds.[121]

Physical Agents and Mechanical Modalities

Whirlpool may be beneficial for Ms. Malloy for several reasons.[86,89,118,121,128-130] It removes loosely adhered debris, bacteria, exudate, and residual topical agents. Whirlpool will hydrate the wound bed, promoting moist wound healing and may decrease the pain associated with wound management techniques. It is preferable to pulsatile lavage due to the small size of the patient's fingers, and whirlpool has the ability to provide an environment that enhances ROM of affected areas.

COORDINATION, COMMUNICATION, AND DOCUMENTATION

Care will be coordinated with Ms. Malloy's son to allow him to assist with wound bandaging. All elements of the patient's management will be documented.

PATIENT/CLIENT-RELATED INSTRUCTION

Ms. Malloy and her son will be instructed in the management of her burns. Particular emphasis will be placed on:

♦ The signs and symptoms of wound infection and action plan if these occur
♦ Proper wound management
♦ Methods to control/minimize scar tissue formation
♦ Because Ms. Malloy's preferred learning style is review of written information, she will be provided with written copies of instructional material, HEP, and self-care techniques

THERAPEUTIC EXERCISE

♦ Flexibility exercises
  ● Exercises are done with each dressing change and a total of two times per day
  ● All AROM exercises will be repeated 10 to 20 times and will include:

  ■ Active gripping of a racquetball ball
  ■ Wringing a dry dish towel
  ■ Active MCP flexion digits 2 to 5, active assisted range of motion (AAROM) digits 3 and 4
  ■ Active PIP flexion digits 2 to 5, AAROM digit 4

FUNCTIONAL TRAINING IN SELF-CARE AND HOME MANAGEMENT

Because a superficial partial-thickness burn can be expected to heal within 10 to 14 days,[131] it was not deemed necessary to adapt her functional activities.

♦ Self-care and home management
  ● The wounds may be left uncovered for showering
  ● A new bandage should be applied afterward
  ● The right hand can be used for dishwashing if a large elbow-length dish glove is worn on the right hand
  ● Ms. Malloy should be encouraged to use the right hand for ADL to help increase AROM and skin extensibility

FUNCTIONAL TRAINING IN WORK, COMMUNITY, AND LEISURE INTEGRATION OR REINTEGRATION

♦ Leisure
  ● Ms. Malloy should be encouraged to return to drawing to assist with regaining functional right hand abilities
  ● If painting, Ms. Malloy should ensure her right hand bandages remain clean and dry
  ● Wearing a thin latex glove on her right hand while painting and a rubber kitchen glove on her right hand while cleaning up may be beneficial

INTEGUMENTARY REPAIR AND PROTECTION TECHNIQUES

♦ Debridement: Selective
  ● Forceps will be used to assist with the removal of any new slough and old topical agents within the wound bed while her hand is in/over the whirlpool
♦ Dressings
  ● The wounds will be covered with a petrolatum-impregnated gauze
  ● Each digit will be wrapped individually with a two-ply roll gauze to decrease dressing bulk and allow increased functional use of the right hand
  ● Dressing change frequency will be decreased to daily
  ● However, if the bandage slides or becomes wet, it will be changed more often
  ● The gauze dressing will be changed to simple adhe-

sive bandages as soon as wound size has decreased to allow coverage of all open areas
- ◆ Topical agents
  - A skin sealant will be applied to the macerated areas and to the periwound skin once maceration has resolved
  - Bacitracin will be applied directly to the wounds using a calcium-alginate swab

PHYSICAL AGENTS AND MECHANICAL MODALITIES

- ◆ Hydrotherapy
  - After removing her dressing, her hand is placed in a whirlpool filled with 92° to 98°F water for 10 minutes
  - During the whirlpool she will perform AROM of the right hand
  - With the whirlpool turbines turned off, the physical therapist will assist with ROM exercises if needed
  - After the whirlpool treatment has been completed, the wounds will be irrigated with normal saline using a 35-mL syringe with a 19-gauge angiocatheter
  - The physical therapist will wear appropriate personal protective equipment, including, but not necessarily limited to, clean gloves, a face shield, hair covering, foot coverings, and a moisture-impermeable gown

ANTICIPATED GOALS AND EXPECTED OUTCOMES

- ◆ Impact on pathology/pathophysiology
  - Pain is reduced to 0/10 in 2 weeks.
  - Periwound maceration is resolved in 1 week.
  - Right hand edema is resolved in 1 week.
  - Tissue perfusion and oxygenation are enhanced.
- ◆ Impact on impairments
  - Integumentary integrity is restored in 2 weeks.
  - Right grip strength is 40 kg without pain in 2 weeks.
  - Right hand AROM is restored to full in 2 weeks.
- ◆ Impact on functional limitations
  - Patient is able to brush her teeth without difficulty in 1 week.
  - Patient is able to return to regular weight training exercises in 1 week.
  - Patient is able to wash, with the use of a latex glove to protect bandages if needed, in 1 week.
  - Patient is able to write with a pen without difficulty in 1 week.
- ◆ Risk reduction/prevention
  - Risk of secondary impairment is reduced.
  - Safety is improved.

- ◆ Impact on health, wellness, and fitness
  - Health status is improved.
  - Physical function is improved.
- ◆ Impact on societal resources
  - Resources are utilized in a cost-effective way.
  - Utilization of physical therapy services is optimized.
- ◆ Patient/client satisfaction
  - Documentation occurs throughout patient management and follows APTA's *Guidelines for Physical Therapy Documentation.*[100]
  - Patient knowledge and awareness of the diagnosis, prognosis, interventions, and anticipated goals and outcomes are increased.
  - Patient understanding of anticipated goals and expected outcomes is increased.

REEXAMINATION

Reexamination is performed throughout the episode of care.

DISCHARGE

Ms. Malloy is discharged from physical therapy after a total of three physical therapy sessions and attainment of her goals and expectations. These sessions have covered her entire episode of care. She is discharged because she has achieved her goals and expected outcomes.

PSYCHOLOGICAL ASPECTS

Because Ms. Malloy is a painter, she is likely to be concerned about the potential to return to activities that require highly skilled use of her right hand. She should be informed of the normal course of healing for a small, superficial partial-thickness burn.[132]

REFERENCES

1. Bates-Jensen BM. Chronic wound assessment. *Nurs Clin North Am.* 1999;34(4):799-845.
2. Carpenter JP. Noninvasive assessment of peripheral vascular occlusive disease. *Advances in Skin and Wound Care.* 2000;13(2):84-85.
3. Blank CA, Irwin GH. Peripheral vascular disorders: assessment and intervention. *Nurs Clin North Am.* 1990;25(4):777-794.
4. Seeley RR, Stephens TD, Tate P. *Anatomy and Physiology.* 5th ed. Boston, Mass: McGraw-Hill Companies; 2000.
5. Ting M. Wound healing and peripheral vascular disease. *Crit Care Nurs Clin North Am.* 1991;3(3):515-523.
6. Rudolph DM. Pathophysiology and management of venous ulcers. *J Wound Ostomy Continence Nurs.* 1998;25(5):248-255.

7. Hess CT. Management of the patient with a venous ulcer. *Advances in Skin and Wound Care.* 2000;13:79-83.

8. Strete D, Creek C. *An Atlas to Human Anatomy.* Boston, Mass: McGraw-Hill; 2000.

9. Hollinworth H. Venous leg ulcers part I: aetiology. *Prof Nurs.* 1998;13(8):555-558.

10. Vander AJ, Sherman JH, Luciano DS. *Human Physiology: The Mechanisms of Body Function.* 5th ed. New York, NY: McGraw-Hill Publishing Co; 1990.

11. Black SB. Venous stasis ulcers: a review. *Ostomy/Wound Management.* 1995;41(8):20-32.

12. Burton CS. Management of chronic and problem lower extremity wounds. *Dermatol Clin.* 1993;11(4):767-773.

13. Moore Z. Compression bandaging: are practitioners achieving the ideal sub-bandage pressures? *J Wound Care.* 2002;11(7):265-268.

14. Applegate EJ. *The Anatomy and Physiology Learning System.* Philadelphia, Pa: WB Saunders Co; 1995.

15. Pecararo RE, Reinber GE, Burgess EM. Pathways to diabetic limb amputation: basis for prevention. *Diabetes Care.* 1990;13:513-521.

16. Cameron J. Arterial leg ulcers. *Nurs Standard.* 1996;10(26):50-56.

17. Doughty DB, Waldrop J, Ramundo J. Lower-extremity ulcers of vascular etiology. In: Bryant RA, ed. *Acute and Chronic Wounds: Nursing Management.* St. Louis, Mo: Mosby; 2000.

18. Greenland P. Clinical significance, detection, and medical treatment for peripheral arterial disease. *J Cardiopulm Rehabil.* 2002;22(2):73-79.

19. Cooke JP, Ma AO. Medical therapy of peripheral arterial occlusive disease. *Surg Clin North Am.* 1995;75(4):569-579.

20. Ouriel K. Peripheral arterial disease. *Lancet.* 2001;358:1257-1264.

21. Beard JD. ABC of arterial and venous disease: chronic lower limb ischaemia. *BMJ.* 2000;320:854-857.

22. Myers BA. *Wound Management: Principles and Practice.* Upper Saddle River, NJ: Prentice Hall; 2004.

23. Lewis CD. Peripheral arterial disease of the lower extremity. *J Cardiovasc Nurs.* 2001;15(4):45-63.

24. Samuelson B, Norton VC. Diagnosis and treatment of peripheral vascular disease: the key in evaluating symptomatic patients is determining if acute life-threatening ischemia is present. *Emerg Med.* 1999;31(12):54-64.

25. Hunt TK, Hopf HW. Wound healing and wound infection: what surgeons and anesthesiologists can do. *Surg Clin North Am.* 1997;77(3):587-606.

26. Orsted HL, Radke L, Gorst R. The impact of musculoskeletal changes on the dynamics of the calf muscle pump. *Ostomy/Wound Management.* 2001;47(10):18-24.

27. Laing P. Diabetic foot ulcers. *Am J Surg.* 1994;167(1A):31S-36S.

28. Kerstein MD, Gahtan V. Outcomes of venous ulcer care: results of a longitudinal study. *Ostomy/Wound Management.* 2000;46(6):22-29.

29. Lippmann HI, Fishman LM, Farrar RH, Bernstein RK, Zybert PA. Edema control in the management of disabling chronic venous insufficiency. *Arch Phys Med Rehabil.* 1994;75:436-441.

30. Carlson MA. Acute wound failure. *Surg Clin North Am.* 1997;77(3):607-636.

31. Eaglstein WH, Falanga V. Chronic wounds. *Surg Clin North Am.* 1997;77(3):689-700.

32. Butler CM, Smith PDC. Microcirculatory aspects of venous ulceration. *J Dermatol Surg Oncol.* 1994;20:474-480.

33. Goodman CC, Boissonault WG. *Pathology: Implications for the Physical Therapist.* Philadelphia, Pa: WB Saunders Co; 1998.

34. Ward K, Schwartz ML, Thiele R, Yoon P. Lower extremity manifestations of vascular disease. *Clin Podiatr Med Surg.* 1998;15(4):629-672.

35. Collins KA, Sumpio BE. Vascular assessment. *Clin Podiatr Med Surg.* 2000;17(2):171-191.

36. Mustafa BO, Rathbun SW, Whitsett TL, Rashkob GE. Sensitivity and specificity of ultrasonography in the diagnosis of upper extremity deep vein thrombosis: a systematic review. *Arch Intern Med.* 2002;162(4):401-404.

37. Powell M, Kirshblum S, O'Connor KC. Duplex ultrasound screening for deep vein thrombosis in spinal cord injured patients at rehabilitation admission. *Arch Phys Med Rehabil.* 1999;80(9):1044-1046.

38. Napodano RJ. Deep vein thrombosis. In: Panzer RJ, Black ER, Grier PF, eds. *Diagnostic Strategies for Common Medical Problems.* Philadelphia, Pa: American College of Physicians; 1991:84-93.

39. Velazquez OC, Baum RA, Carpenter JP. Magnetic resonance angiography of lower extremity arterial disease. *Surg Clin North Am.* 1998;78(4):519-537.

40. Koelemay M, Lijmer J, Legemate D, Bossuyt P. Magnetic resonance angiography for the evaluation of lower extremity arterial disease: a meta-analysis. *JAMA.* 2001;285(10):1338-1345.

41. Kominsky SJ. *Medical and Surgical Management of the Diabetic Foot.* St. Louis, Mo: Mosby-Year Book, Inc; 1994.

42. American Diabetes Association. Consensus development conference on diabetic foot care. *Diabetes Care.* 1999;22(8):1354-1360.

43. American Diabetes Association. Peripheral arterial disease in people with diabetes. *Diabetes Care.* 2003;26(12):3333-3341.

44. Benowitz NL. Antihypertensive agents. In: Katzung BG, ed. *Basic and Clinical Pharmacology.* 8th ed. New York, NY: Lange Medical Books/McGraw-Hill; 2001:155-180.

45. Hoffman BB, Carruthers SG. Cardiovascular disorders: hypertension. In: Carruthers SG, Hoffman BB, Melmon KL, Nierenberg DW, eds. *Melmon and Morrelli's Clinical Pharmacology.* 4th ed. New York, NY: McGraw-Hill; 2000:114-130.

46. Crouse J, Allan M, Elam M. Clinical manifestation of atherosclerotic peripheral arterial disease and the role of cilostazol in treatment of intermittent claudication. *J Clin Pharmacol.* 2002;42:1291-1298.

47. Jull A, Waters J, Arrol B. Pentoxifyline for treating venous leg ulcers (Cochrane review). *The Cochrane Library.* 2002(2), Oxford, Update software.

48. Falanga V, Fujitana RM, Diaz C, et al. Systemic treatment of venous leg ulcers with high doses of pentoxyfylline: efficacy in a randomized, placebo-controlled trial. *Wound Repair Regen.* 1999;7(4):208-213.

49. Whitselt TL. Peripheral arterial occlusive disease. In: Carruthers SG, Hoffman BB, Melmon KL, Nierenberg DW, eds. *Melmon and Morrelli's Clinical Pharmacology.* 4th ed. New York, NY: McGraw-Hill; 2000.

50. Rubano JJ, Kerstein MD. Arterial insufficiency and vasculitides. *J Wound Ostomy Continence Nurs.* 1998;25(3):147-157.

51. Sibbald RG. Venous leg ulcers. *Ostomy/Wound Management.* 1998;44(9):52-64.

52. Adler PF. Assessing the effects of pentoxifylline (Trental) on diabetic neuropathic foot ulcers. *J Foot Ankle Surg.* 1991;30(3):300-303.

53. Reuters. Dalteparin treatment improves healing of diabetic foot ulcers. *Diabetes Care.* 2003;26:2575-2580, 2689.

54. Malloy MJ, Kane JP. Agents used in hyperlipidemia. In: Benowitz NL, ed. *Basic and Clinical Pharmacology.* New York, NY: Lange Medical Books/McGraw-Hill; 2001:581-595.

55. Franklin BA, ed. *American College of Sports Medicine's Guidelines for Exercise Testing and Prescription.* 6th ed. Philadelphia, Pa: Lippincott Williams & Wilkins; 2000.

56. Schriger D, Baraff L. Defining normal capillary refill: variation with age, sex, and temperature. *Ann Emerg Med.* 1988;17(9):932-935.

57. Strozik K, Pieper C, Cools F. Capillary refill time in newborns—optimal pressing time, site of testing and normal values. *Acta Paediatr.* 1998;87(3):310-312.

58. Gorelick MH, Shaw KN, Murphy KO. Validity and reliability of clinical signs in the diagnosis of dehydration in children. *Pediatrics.* 1997;99(5):e6.

59. McGee SR, Boyko EJ. Physical examination and chronic lower-extremity ischemia: a critical review. *Arch Intern Med.* 1998;158:1357-1364.

60. Fiegelson H, Criqui MH, Fronek A, Langer R, Molgaard C. Screening for peripheral arterial disease: the sensitivity, specificity, and predictive value of noninvasive tests in a defined population. *Am J Epidemiol.* 1994;140(6):426-534.

61. Leng G, Fowkes F, Lee A, Dunbar J, Housley E, Ruckey C. Use of ankle brachial pressure index to predict cardiovascular events and death: a cohort study. *BMJ.* 1996;313:1440-1443.

62. Cantwell-Gab K. Identifying chronic peripheral arterial disease. *Am J Nurs.* 1996;96(7):40-47.

63. Sloan H, Wills EM. Ankle-brachial index: calculating your patient's vascular risk. *Nursing.* 1999;29(10):58-59.

64. Jaffe MR. Diagnosis of peripheral arterial disease: utility of the vascular laboratory. *Clin Cornerstone.* 2002;4(5).

65. Dillavou E, Kahn MB. Peripheral vascular disease: diagnosing and treating the three most common peripheral vasculopathies. *Geriatrics.* 2003;58(2):37-42.

66. Magee DJ. *Orthopedic Physical Assessment.* 3rd ed. Philadelphia, Pa: WB Saunders Co; 1997:638.

67. Urbano F. Homans' sign in the diagnosis of deep vein thrombosis. *Hosp Phys.* 2001;March:22-24.

68. Anand SS, Wells PS, Hunt D, Brill-Edwards P, Cook D, Ginsberg JS. Does this patient have a deep vein thrombosis? *JAMA.* 1998;279(14):1094-1099.

69. Ofri D. Diagnosis and treatment of deep vein thrombosis. *West J Med.* 2000;173:194-197.

70. Ferraz M, Quaresma M, Aquino L, Atra E, Tugwell P, Goldsmith C. Reliability of pain scales in the assessment of literate and illiterate patients with rheumatoid arthritis. *J Rheumatol.* 1990;17(8):1022-1024.

71. Hoher J, Munster A, Klein J, Eypasch E, Tilling T. Validation and application of a subjective knee questionnaire. *Knee Surg Sports Traumatol Arthrosc.* 1995;3(1):26-33.

72. Paice JA, Cohen FL. Validity of a verbally administered numeric rating scale to measure cancer pain intensity. *Cancer Nurs.* 1997;20(2):88-93.

73. Poore S, Cameron J. Venous leg ulcer recurrence: prevention and healing. *J Wound Care.* 2002;11(5):197-199.

74. McGuckin M, Williams L, Brooks J, Cherry GW. Guidelines in practice: the effect on healing of venous ulcers. *Advances in Skin and Wound Care.* 2001;14(1):33-36.

75. Cullum N, Nelson E, Fletcher AW, Sheldon TA. Compression for venous leg ulcers (Cochrane review). *The Cochrane Library.* 2002(2).

76. Bergan JJ, Sparks SR. Non-elastic compression: an alternative in management of chronic venous insufficiency. *J Wound Ostomy Continence Nurs.* 2000;27(2):83-89.

77. Nelson E, Bell-Syer S, et al. Compression for preventing recurrence of venous ulcers. *The Cochrane Library.* 2000(2).

78. Sieggreen MY, Maklebust J. Debridement: choices and challenges. *Advances in Skin and Wound Care.* 1997;10(2):32-37.

79. Singhal K, Reis G, Kerstein MD. Options for nonsurgical debridement of necrotic wounds. *Advances in Skin and Wound Care.* 2001;14(2):96-103.

80. Enoch S, Harding K. Wound bed preparation: the science behind the removal of barriers to healing. *Wounds.* 2003;15(7):213-229.

81. Ovington LG. Wound care products: how to choose. *Advances in Skin and Wound Care.* 2001;14(5):224-232.

82. Bolton LL, Monte K, Pirone LA. Moisture and healing: beyond the jargon. *Ostomy/Wound Management.* 2000;46(1A):51S-62S.

83. Sprung P, Hou Z, Ladin DA. Hydrogels and hydrocolloids: an objective product comparison. *Ostomy/Wound Management.* 1998;44(1):36-53.

84. Morgan D, Hoelscher J. Pulsed lavage: promoting comfort and healing in home care. *Ostomy/Wound Management.* 2000;46(4):44-49.

85. Luedtke-Hoffman K, Shafer DS. Pulsed lavage in wound cleansing. *Phys Ther.* 2000;80(3):292-300.

86. Barr JE. Principles of wound cleansing. *Ostomy/Wound Management.* 1995;41(7A):15S-22S.

87. Loehne HB. Pulsatile lavage with concurrent suction. In: Sussman C, Bates-Jensen BM, eds. *Wound Care: A Collaborative Practice Manual for Physical Therapists and Nurses.* 2nd ed. Gaithersburg, Md: Aspen Publications; 2001:643-660.

88. Scott RG, Loehne HB. Treatment options: 5 questions and answers about pulsed lavage. *Advances in Skin and Wound Care.* 2000;13(3):133-134.

89. McCulloch JM. Physical modalities in wound management: ultrasound, vasopneumatic devices, hydrotherapy. *Ostomy/Wound Management.* 1995;41(5):30-37.

90. McCulloch J, Boyd VB. The effects of whirlpool and dependent position on lower extremity volume. *J Orthop Sports Phys Ther.* 1992;16(4):169-173.

91. Haynes L, Brown M, Handley B, et al. PO-012-M: comparison of Pulsavac and sterile whirlpool regarding the promotion of tissue granulation. *Phys Ther.* 1994;64(5):S4.

92. Reichardt LE. Venous ulceration: compression as the mainstay of therapy. *J Wound Ostomy Continence Nurs.* 1999;26:39-47.

93. Marston W, et al. Healing rates and cost efficacy of outpatient compression treatment for leg ulcers associated with venous insufficiency. *J Vasc Surg.* 1999;30(3):491-498.

94. Stotts NA, Wipke-Tevis D. Co-factors in impaired healing. *Ostomy/Wound Management*. 1996;42(2):44-53.

95. Center FCI. The Food Guide Pyramid [web page]. 1996. Available att: http://www.pueblo.gsa.gov/cic_text/food/food-pyramind/main/htm. Accessed August 25, 2004.

96. Ayello EA, Thomas DR, Litchford MA. Nutritional aspects of wound healing. *Home Healthcare Nurs*. 1999;17(11):719-729.

97. Cohn JC, Lowry A. It's all in the stocking. *Rehab Management*. 2002;15(5):36-40.

98. Alexander D, Gammage D, Nichols A, Gaskins D. Analysis of strike-through contamination in saturated sterile dressings. *Clin Nurs Res*. 1992;1(1):28-34.

99. Popovich DM, Alexander D, Martorella C, Jackson L. Strike-through contamination in saturated sterile dressings: a clinical analysis. *Clin Nurs Res*. 1995;4(2):195-207.

100. American Physical Therapy Association. Guide to physical therapist practice. 2nd ed. *Phys Ther*. 2001;81:9-744.

101. Tinetti ME. Performance oriented assessment of mobility problems in elderly patients. *J Am Geriatr Soc*. 1986;34(2):119-126.

102. VanSwearingen JM, Brach JS. Making geriatric assessment work: selecting useful measures. *Phys Ther*. 2001;81:1233-1252.

103. Tinetti ME, Williams TF, Mayewski R. Fall risk index for elderly patients based on number of chronic disabilities. *Am J Med*. 1986;80:429-434.

104. Harada N, Chiu V, Damron-Rodriguez J, Fowler E, Siu A, Reuben DB. Screening for balance and mobility impairment in elderly individuals living in residential care facilities. *Phys Ther*. 1995;75:462-469.

105. Steffen TM, Hacker TA, Mollinger L. Age-and gender-related test performance in community-dwelling elderly people: six-minute walk test, Berg balance scale, timed up and go test, and gait speeds. *Phys Ther*. 2002;82:128-137.

106. Thornbahn L, Newton R. Use of the Berg balance test to predict falls in elderly persons. *Phys Ther*. 1996;76(6):576-585.

107. Maklebust J. Interrupting the pressure ulcer cycle. *Nurs Clin North Am*. 1999;34(4):861-872.

108. Bergstrom N, Braden BJ, Kemp MG, Champagne M, Ruby E. Predicting pressure ulcer risk: a multi-site study of the predictive validity of the Braden scale. *Nurs Res*. 1998;47(5):261-269.

109. Bandy W, Irion J. The effect of time on static stretching on the flexibility of hamstring muscles. *Phys Ther*. 1994;74(9):845-852.

110. Bergstrom N, Bennett MA, Carlson CE, et al. Treatment of Pressure Ulcers: Clinical Practice Guideline No. 15. Rockville, Md: US Department of Health and Human Services. Agency for Health Care Policy and Research; December 1994. AHCPR Publication No. 95-0652.

111. Maklebust J. Using wound care products to promote a healing environment. *Crit Care Nurs Clin North Am*. 1996;8(2):141-158.

112. McCulloch JM. Decision point: wound dressings. *PT Magazine*. 1996;4(5):52-62.

113. Kraft MR, Lawson L, Pohlmann B, Reid-Lokos C, Barder L. A comparison of Epilock and saline dressings in the treatment of pressure ulcers. *Decubitus*. 1993;6(6):42-48.

114. Barr JE. Multi-center evaluation of a new wound dressing. *Ostomy/Wound Management*. 1993;39(9):60-67.

115. Sibbald RG, Williamson D, Osrsted HL, et al. Preparing the wound bed: debridement, bacterial balance, and moisture balance. *Ostomy/Wound Management*. 2000;46(11):14-35.

116. Sheridan RL. Evaluating and managing burn wounds. *Dermatol Clin*. 2000;12(1):17-28.

117. Richard R. Assessment and diagnosis of burn wounds. *Advances in Skin and Wound Care*. 1999;12(9):468-471.

118. Staley M, Richard R. Management of the acute burn wound: an overview. *Advances in Skin and Wound Care*. 1997;10(2):39-44.

119. McCain D, Sutherland S. Nursing essentials: skin grafts for patient with burns. *Am J Nurs*. 1998;98(7):34-49.

120. Pessina MA, Ellis SM. Rehabilitation. *Nurs Clin North Am*. 1997;32(2):365-372.

121. Howell JW. Management of the acutely burned hand for the nonspecialized clinician. *Phys Ther*. 1989;69(12):1077-1090.

122. Bohannon RW. Whirlpool versus whirlpool and rinse for removal of bacteria from a venous stasis ulcer. *Phys Ther*. 1982;62(3):304-308.

123. Jordon BS, Harrington DJ. Management of the burn wound. *Nurs Clin North Am*. 1997;32(2):251-273.

124. Ward RS, Saffle JR. Topical agents in burn and wound care. *Phys Ther*. 1995;75(6):526-538.

125. Evans RB. An update on wound management. *Frontiers Hand Rehabil*. 1991;7(3):409-432.

126. Wiseman DM, Rovee DT, Alvarez OM. Wound dressings: design and use. In: Cohen IK, Diegelmann RF, Lindbald WJ, eds. *Wound Healing: Biochemical and Clinical Aspects*. Philadelphia, Pa: WB Saunders Co; 1992.

127. Brown-Etris M, Smith JA, Pasceri P, Punchello M. Case studies: considering dressing options. *Ostomy/Wound Management*. 1994;40(5):46-53.

128. Feedar JA. Physical therapy modalities to augment wound healing. *Top Geriatr Rehabil*. 1994;9(4):43-57.

129. Shankowsky HA, Callioux LS, Tredget E. North American survey of hydrotherapy in modern burn care. *J Burn Care Rehabil*. 1994;15:143-146.

130. Burke DT, Ho C, Saucier MA, Stewart G. Effects of hydrotherapy on pressure ulcer healing. *Am J Phys Med Rehabil*. 1998;77(5):394-398.

131. Mertens DM, Jenkins ME, Warden GD. Out-patient burn management. *Nurs Clin North Am*. 1997;32(2):343-364.

132. Davis ST, Sheely-Adolphson P. Psychosocial interventions: pharmacologic and psychologic modalities. *Nurs Clin North Am*. 1997;32(2):331-342.

CHAPTER FOUR

Impaired Integumentary Integrity Associated With Full-Thickness Skin Involvement and Scar Formation (Pattern D)

Betsy A. Myers, PT, MPT, MHS, OCS, CLT

INTRODUCTION

Full-thickness wounds involve the epidermis, dermis, and the subcutaneous tissues, but not the fascial plane. Examples of full-thickness wounds include Stage III pressure ulcers (see Table 2-7), Wagner Grade 1 (see Table 2-2) neuropathic ulcers, full-thickness (or third-degree) burns, and some wounds due to surgery, vascular insufficiency, or trauma. Neuropathic ulcers may range in depth from superficial skin involvement (Pattern B: Impaired Integumentary Integrity Associated With Superficial Skin Involvement) to full-thickness extending into fascia, muscle, or bone (Pattern E: Impaired Integumentary Integrity Associated With Skin Involvement Extending Into Fascia, Muscle, or Bone and Scar Formation). However, the majority of neuropathic ulcerations that require physical therapy interventions will have partial-thickness (Pattern C: Impaired Integumentary Integrity Associated With Partial-Thickness Skin Involvement and Scar Formation) or full-thickness (Pattern D: Impaired Integumentary Integrity Associated With Full-Thickness Skin Involvement and Scar Formation) skin involvement.[1]

ANATOMY

The anatomy and physiology of the skin has been reviewed in Pattern A: Primary Prevention/Risk Reduction for Integumentary Disorders. Since many of the ulcers in this pattern are the result of diabetes, the anatomy and physiology will concentrate on the structures involved in maintaining the body's blood sugar levels. Normal blood sugar concentration ranges between 70 to 110 mg/dL.[2] Euglycemia is maintained through a delicate balance between glucose storage and production that is controlled by the complex interaction between the pancreas, the liver, muscle tissue, and adipose tissue.

The pancreas consists of two major types of cells: acini and islets of Langerhans. The acini secrete enzymes into the intestine to aide in digestion and are not directly involved in blood sugar regulation. The islets of Langerhans secrete three different hormones into the bloodstream. The alpha cells secrete glucagon that helps to increase the blood sugar level. The beta cells secrete insulin that facilitates glucose transport into body cells and lowers blood sugar concentrations. The delta cells secrete somatostatin that inhibits the release of glucagon and insulin and decreases gastrointestinal activity to extend the time in which nutrients are absorbed.[2]

PHYSIOLOGY

The central and peripheral nervous systems require a constant supply of glucose to fuel their energy needs. In contrast, although muscle tissue, adipose tissue, and the liver are able to use glucose for energy, they rely primarily on glycogen

Insulin

Liver	Muscle	Adipose
↑ glucose storage	↑ protein synthesis	↑ transport of fatty acids
Inhibits gluconeogenesis synthesis	↑ glucose uptake	↑ triglycerides

Figure 4-1. Insulin lowers blood glucose levels by acting on the liver, muscle, and adipose tissue.

and fatty acids for energy. After eating a meal, there is a rise in blood glucose levels, some of which is used to maintain normal blood sugar concentrations to allow adequate energy substrates for the nervous system. However, the majority is removed from the bloodstream and stored for future use as glycogen or converted into fat.[2]

The rise in blood sugar levels stimulates the release of insulin from pancreatic beta cells to lower blood sugar levels to within the normal range. Insulin, also known as the building and storing hormone, is formed by the cleavage of a larger proinsulin protein into the biologically active insulin, composed of linked A and B chains, and the biologically inactive, but clinically measurable, C-peptide chain. The active form of insulin is able to bind with insulin receptors that increase the transport of glucose into body cells lowering blood glucose levels. Insulin acts on the liver to increase the storage of glucose in the form of glycogen and to inhibit gluconeogenesis, the conversion of glycogen into glucose. Insulin acts on muscle tissue to increase the transport of amino acids into cells and increase protein synthesis. Insulin acts on adipose tissue to increase the transport of fatty acid into cells and increase triglyceride synthesis (Figure 4-1).[2,3]

The decline in blood sugar levels that occurs between meals stimulates the alpha cells to release glucagon. The actions of glucagon oppose those of insulin (Table 4-1). Glucagon increases the breakdown of glycogen (glycogenolysis) and promotes the formation of glucose (gluconeogenesis) by the liver. Glucagon acts on adipose tissue to increase the breakdown of fat into fatty acids and glycerol, a substrate

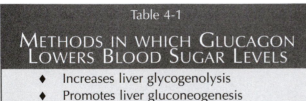

Table 4-1

METHODS IN WHICH GLUCAGON LOWERS BLOOD SUGAR LEVELS

- ♦ Increases liver glycogenolysis
- ♦ Promotes liver gluconeogenesis
- ♦ Increases the breakdown of fat
- ♦ Increases the breakdown of protein

for gluconeogenesis. Glucagon increases the breakdown of protein into amino acids and then into glucose precursors. Hypoglycemia also stimulates the sympathetic nervous system causing the hypothalamic-pituitary-adrenal release of growth hormone, cortisol, and epinephrine. Collectively referred to as counter-regulatory hormones, these three hormones act to increase glycogenolysis and inhibit insulin release.[4]

PATHOPHYSIOLOGY

Diabetes is a disorder of glucose, protein, and fat metabolism related to alterations in the body's ability to produce or use insulin. There are several types and subtypes of diabetes mellitus. However, the majority of individuals who will be seen within the physical therapy setting have Type 1A or Type 2 diabetes. Patients with type I diabetes are incapable of making insulin.[3] Type 1A diabetes, formerly known as juvenile diabetes or IDDM, is typically diagnosed in children and young adults and is believed to be immune-mediated. There is a genetic predisposition for developing Type 1 diabetes with a 5% chance of developing diabetes if one parent has Type 1 diabetes and a 20% chance if both parents have Type 1 diabetes. In addition, researchers believe there may be an environmental trigger for the development of Type 1A diabetes. Type 1B, or idiopathic, diabetes represents a fraction of individuals with Type 1 diabetes and appears to be strongly hereditary. Most individuals with Type 1B diabetes are of African or Asian descent. Because patients with Type 1 diabetes do not produce insulin, they require exogenous insulin replacement therapy to lower blood glucose levels, to regulate metabolism of fats and protein, and to prevent ketosis. Individuals with Type 1 diabetes comprise approximately 10% of all patients with diabetes.[2,5]

In contrast, patients with Type 2 diabetes have impaired insulin secretion or insulin insensitivity.[3] Individuals with Type 2 diabetes are typically diagnosed at middle age or later and approximately 80% are overweight.[2] The exact cause of Type 2 diabetes is unknown. Although it is not immune-mediated, there may be a genetic predisposition to developing Type 2 diabetes. Other proposed causes of Type 2 diabetes are the development of insulin resistance; impaired insulin secretion; beta cell defects causing the body to make a slightly altered, less active version of insulin; and certain health behaviors such as inactivity, poor diet, and obesity.[6] Patients with Type 2 diabetes make up approximately 90% of all individuals with diabetes, or approximately 16 million Americans, and a majority of amputations are due to long-term complications of diabetes.[7]

There are three hypotheses as to the mechanism by which the sustained hyperglycemia of diabetes leads to tissue damage.

1. Tissue damage may be due to hemodynamic changes caused by sustained hyperglycemia and the resultant changes in microvascular pressures.[8]

2. The structural changes of proteins bound to glucose, or chemical reactions with these structures, may cause tissue trauma either directly, or indirectly, by the formation of free radicals.[9]

3. The breakdown of glucose through the polyol pathway leads to an accumulation of sorbitol that may result in tissue destruction.[10-12]

Approximately 15% of individuals with diabetes have had an ulcer on the foot or ankle.[13] Diabetes is thought to be the primary causative factor in 45% of all LE amputations.[14] A retrospective record review of patients with diabetes in a large health maintenance organization demonstrated a 5.8% incidence of neuropathic ulcerations. Of these, 15% developed osteomyelitis and 15.6% required amputation. The 3-year survival rate for patients with ulcers was 13% less than for patients without ulcers.[15]

Many risk factors may contribute to neuropathic ulceration and delayed wound healing. Arguably the single greatest risk factor for ulceration in patients with diabetes is neuropathy.[16,17] Neuropathy is the most common complication of diabetes and may include sensory, motor, and/or autonomic dysfunction. Sensory neuropathy is the loss of protective sensation, defined as being unable to detect a size 5.07 Semmes-Weinstein monofilament.[18-21] Eight percent of patients with diabetes were found to have sensory neuropathy at the time of diagnosis, whereas 50% were found to have sensory neuropathy 25 years after initial diagnosis.[7] Because sensory loss is gradual and often painless, patients may be unaware of trauma as minor as a blister from poorly fitted shoes or as significant as a shard of glass embedded in the foot until either visually inspecting their feet or signs of infection become apparent. Motor neuropathy leads to intrinsic muscle wasting and may predispose patients with diabetes to plantar ulceration by the resulting increase in plantar pressures and shear forces.[22,23] Autonomic neuropathy may predispose patients with diabetes to ulcerations in four ways.[13]

1. It causes an alteration in the body's ability to sweat leading to dry, inelastic, and cracked skin allowing microbes a pathway to enter the body.

2. Autonomic neuropathy leads to an increased rate of callus formation, producing localized areas of increased pressure.

3. Autonomic neuropathy may lead to arteriovenous shunting resulting in decreased perfusion of the skin and decreased potential for tissue repair.

4. Autonomic neuropathy leads to hyperperfusion of bone, which essentially leaches the bone of calcium, predisposing the bones of the foot to osteopenic fracture.[24]

Diabetes accelerates the rate of atherosclerosis and is the leading risk factor for peripheral vascular disease. Diabetes may cause thickening of the basement membrane, presumably decreasing the exchange of oxygen and nutrients in affected vessels. Individuals with diabetes who smoke are at an even greater risk for peripheral vascular disease.[25] Mechanical stress due to abnormal or excessive forces places the individual with diabetes at risk for ulceration. Therefore, individuals with foot deformities or limited foot mobility should be considered at risk for ulceration.[1] Individuals with diabetes, particularly those with sensory neuropathy, who choose to walk barefoot or with inadequate footwear are at risk for ulceration due to undetected trauma. Diabetes is the leading cause of blindness due to retinopathy, glaucoma, and cataracts.[2] Nearly all of patients with Type 1 diabetes and over half of those with Type 2 diabetes were found to have some degree of retinopathy 20 years after their initial diagnosis.[26] Decreased vision, in combination with neuropathy, further inhibits early recognition of skin trauma in patients with diabetes.

Sustained hyperglycemia decreases all three phases of wound healing and the body's ability to fight infection.[5] High blood sugar levels decrease the rate of collagen synthesis, angiogenesis, and fibroblast proliferation and reduce the tensile strength of incisional wounds. In addition, high blood sugar levels impair granulocyte chemotaxis phagocytosis and opsonization of bacteria.[27] The Diabetes Control and Complications Trial, the United Kingdom Prospective Diabetes Study Group, and several smaller group studies clearly demonstrate that the development and progression of long-term complications affecting wound healing, including neuropathy, retinopathy, vascular disease, and decreased ability to fight infection, can be slowed or reversed with improvements in glycemic control.[28,29] Therefore, once an ulceration occurs, aggressive wound management interventions along with education and methods to improve glycemic control should be initiated immediately to maximize wound healing and prevent serious complications.

Neuropathic ulcers have some characteristic features (Table 4-2). They are located on the plantar aspect of the foot, primarily in areas of increased pressure or shear forces or in areas of trauma. They typically appear as round punched-out lesions with a callused rim. Neuropathic ulcers are generally free of necrotic tissue except in the presence of arterial insufficiency or infection. The integumentary changes may include: anhydrous, callused skin; thickening of the toenails due to fungal infection; and structural changes of the foot, such as Charcot foot, clawing of the toes, or prior ulceration/amputation. Vasodilation due to autonomic neuropathy may lead to peripheral edema and a mild increase in tissue temperature even without the presence of infection. Neuropathic ulcerations are typically painless due to sensory neuropathy, however, some patients may report paresthesias.[1,27]

IMAGING/CLINICAL TESTS

Patients with neuropathic ulcers have an increased risk of infection and an impaired immune response. Neuropathic

Table 4-2
TYPICAL CHARACTERISTICS OF NEUROPATHIC ULCERS

Location	Plantar aspect of the foot
	Areas of trauma on the foot
Pain	Painless
	Lack of protection sensation
Wound	Round, punched-out lesion
	Callus rim
	Granular bed
Other	Anhydrous skin
	Charcot foot
	Clawed toes
	Fungal infections of the toenails
	Prior ulceration/amputation
	Potential for silent infection

ulcerations also tend to be chronic[1] and may be present for several months or even years. Therefore, these wounds may not exhibit the classic signs of wound infection[1] redness, warmth, swelling, and excessive or purulent drainage. A wound culture and sensitivity is able to identify the presence of infection and allows for microbe identification to enable appropriate antimicrobial therapy (see Pattern B: Impaired Integumentary Integrity Associated With Superficial Skin Involvement). Cultures of neuropathic ulcerations typically reveal polymicrobial infections[20] with an average of four to five different microbes, the most common being *Staphylococcus aureus*. Patients with neuropathic ulcerations that have not healed in 4 weeks is cause for concern[1] and should be further assessed for a "silent" infection. Patients with wounds that present with exposed joint capsule or bone should be assessed for the presence of osteomyelitis.[1,30]

The following imaging techniques may be utilized to clarify pathology and to assist with treatment planning.
- ◆ Radiographs
  - Used to identify neuropathic fractures, Charcot foot, and osteomyelitis[1]
  - Radiographs usually cannot detect acute osteomyelitis[30]
  - A clinically stable patient with two negative radiographs that are taken 2 weeks apart is unlikely to have osteomyelitis
  - If the radiograph shows cortical bone erosion, osteomyelitis is probable[1]
  - Radiographic evidence of osteomyelitis may not be evident until approximately 50% of bone mass has been lost[31]
- ◆ Bone scan: Considered to be the gold standard for identifying osteomyelitis[20,30,32]
- ◆ Magnetic resonance imaging (MRI): Has been found

to have good sensitivity and specificity for identifying osteomyelitis in patients with diabetes mellitus[30]

The following clinical tests may be utilized to clarify pathology, to determine a patient's healing potential, and to assist with treatment planning.
- ◆ Swab culture[1,33-36] (Table 4-3)
  - Is used to identify the number and type of organisms present in a wound without traumatizing wound bed or performing surgery
  - A wound is considered infected if microbe concentrations are greater than 10^5 organisms per gram of tissue
- ◆ Tissue biopsy[1,33] (Table 4-4)
  - Is the gold standard for identification of wound infection and the type of offending organism(s)
  - Allows for appropriate treatment, including antimicrobial therapy and/or surgical debridement
- ◆ Fluid aspiration
  - Is used as an alternate method for diagnosing wound infection in which a physician uses a needle to draw 1.0 mL of fluid from within the wound area for laboratory analysis
  - The limitations of fluid aspiration are that it requires sufficient wound fluid for aspiration and is dependent on the skills of the physician
  - Possible complications include infections along the needle tract, fistula formation, and trauma to underlying structures

PHARMACOLOGY

The following pharmacological agents may be utilized in the management of patients with neuropathic ulcerations.
- ◆ Insulin
  - Examples: Regular, NPH, lispro, combination drugs
  - Action: Synthetic form of human insulin
  - Administered: Injection
  - Side effects: Hypoglycemia, hyperglycemia
- ◆ Sulfonylureas[4]
  - Examples: Glyburide, chlorpropamide, tolbutamide, glimepiride
  - Action: Stimulates insulin release from pancreatic beta cells
  - Administered: Oral
  - Side effects: Hypoglycemia, gastrointestinal symptoms
- ◆ Biguanides[4]
  - Examples: Metformin, phenformin
  - Action: Inhibit liver glucose production
  - Administered: Oral
  - Side effects: Hypoglycemia, gastrointestinal symptoms

- Thiazolidase inhibitors[3]
  - Examples: Rosiglitazone, pioglitazone
  - Actions: Decrease hepatic gluconeogenesis, decrease insulin resistance by increasing glucose uptake and metabolism in muscle and adipose tissue
  - Administered: Oral
  - Side effects: Headaches, myalgia, hypoglycemia, hyperglycemia
- Alpha-glucosidase inhibitors[4]
  - Examples: Acarbose, miglitol
  - Actions: Delay the digestion of complex carbohydrates resulting in a smaller rise in blood sugar after eating
  - Administered: Oral
  - Side effects: Gastrointestinal symptoms
- Antibiotics[1]
  - For patients with non-limb-threatening infections
    - Use oral antibiotics that cover the usual offending bacteria (aerobic gram-positive *cocci* such as *Staphylococcus aureus*) but are not too broad spectrum to prevent development of resistant strains of bacteria

- After microbe identification antibiotic should be refined to culture-specific agent
- Examples: Cephalexin, clindamycin, amoxicillin/clavulanate
  - Newer fluoroquinolones, such as trovafloxin, may be used with polymicrobial infections
- Administered: Oral
- Side effects: Gastrointestinal symptoms, skin rash
- For patients with limb-threatening infections
  - Use parenteral antibiotics that are broad spectrum and specific to culture
  - Examples: Vancomycin/ampicillin/sulbactam or piperacillin/tazobactam
  - Administered: Parenteral
  - Side effects: Gastrointestinal symptoms, rash, see appropriate pharmacology text to address specific medications and their side effects
- Osteomyelitis treatment
  - Surgical debridement of bone or infected portion of bone and a long course (>6 weeks) of antibiotics, with 1 to 2 weeks of parenteral treatment

Table 4-3
SWAB CULTURE

Purpose	To identify the number and type of organisms present in a wound
Method	A swab is moved in a 10-point pattern along the viable portions of a wound bed and within tunnels with enough force to express wound fluid
	Swab cultures are sent to a laboratory for analysis
	Aerobic cultures identify oxygen-metabolizing microbes and anaerobic cultures are used to identify non-oxygen dependent microbes
Interpretation	A wound is considered infected if microbe concentrations are greater than 10^5 organisms per gram of tissue
Advantages	May be performed by nonphysician health care professionals
	Noninvasive, quick, painless
Limitations	Primarily samples the wound surface and results may not be as reliable or valid an indicator of infection as a tissue biopsy

Table 4-4
TISSUE BIOPSY

Purpose	To identify a wound infection and the nature of the offending organism(s)
Method	A sample of living tissue is removed during debridement by a physician or podiatrist
	For a bone biopsy, a physician or podiatrist removes a piece of bone percutaneously or during debridement to diagnose the presence or absence of osteomyelitis
Interpretation	Tissue sample is sent to a laboratory for analysis to identify the presence and type of organism
Advantages	Valid and reliable test for diagnosing wound infection
Limitations	Surgical procedure performed by a physician or podiatrist
	Traumatizes wound bed because it requires a sample of living tissue

- Administered: Parenteral
- Side effects: Gastrointestinal symptoms, rash, see appropriate pharmacology text to address specific medications and their side effects

◆ Topical antimicrobials (ointments)
- Examples: Gentamicin, bacitracin, Betadine
- Actions: Inhibit bacterial growth
- Side effects:
  - Hypersensitivity reactions, secondary infections, nephrotoxicity, and ototoxicity
  - As above nephrotoxicity and ototoxicity are rare unless utilized in large volumes

◆ Topical antimicrobials (creams)
- Examples: Silver sulfadiazine, mafenide acetate, nitrofurazone, nystatin
- Actions: Inhibit bacterial and fungal growth
- Side effects: Hypersensitivity reactions, leukopenia, secondary infections

◆ Topical antimicrobials (solutions)
- Examples: Silver nitrate, acetic acid, sodium hypochlorite, mafenide acetate, bacitracin (many of these preparations will need to be made in the institution's pharmacy based on patient need and physician preference)
- Actions: Inhibit bacterial growth
- Side effects: Hypersensitivity reactions, acidosis

Case Study #1:
Full-Thickness Neuropathic Wound

Ms. Edwina Donovan is a 38-year-old female who has a wound on the plantar aspect of her right great toe (Figure 4-2).

PHYSICAL THERAPIST EXAMINATION

HISTORY

◆ General demographics: Ms. Donovan is a 38-year-old female whose primary language is English. She is right-hand dominant. She is a high school graduate.

◆ Social history: She is single and has no children. Her family lives in town.

◆ Employment/work: She works part-time as a technician, which requires sitting while assembling small parts.

◆ Living environment: Ms. Donovan lives alone in a ground-level apartment.

◆ General health status

- General health perception: Ms. Donovan reports that her health status is good.
- Physical function: She reports that her physical function is not limited.
- Psychological function: Normal.
- Role function: Sister, daughter, aunt, self-supporting assembly technician.
- Social function: She enjoys playing cards two nights per week with her family.

◆ Social/health habits: Ms. Donovan is a nondrinker. She smoked one-and-a-half packs of cigarettes per day for 8 years until she quit approximately 2 years ago, However, she restarted smoking a year ago and now smokes two to four cigarettes per day.

◆ Family history: She reports her mother was diagnosed with Type 2 diabetes about 10 years ago, and her father had a heart attack 6 years ago. One sister has Type 2 diabetes. She reports most of her family is overweight.

◆ Medical/surgical history: Ms. Donovan has Type 2 diabetes mellitus and had the distal phalanx of her right great toe amputated 2 years ago after developing a non-healing ulcer. She reports she tests her blood sugar about once a week or so, and it is usually around 250 mg/dL.

◆ Current condition(s)/chief complaint(s): She reports that she noticed what she thought was a blister on the bottom of her great toe about 6 days ago. However, when she got out of the shower yesterday, she thought the wound appeared worse, so she went to the emergency department. She has been covering the wound with an adhesive bandage for the past 3 days.

◆ Functional status and activity level: Ms. Donovan reports that she has no functional limitations. She has never exercised regularly.

◆ Medications: Insulin, metformin.

◆ Other clinical tests: Her chart from the emergency room is available for review (see Table 3-10 for laboratory reference values).

- Hgb=12.0 g/dL
- Hct=31%
- White blood cell count (WBC)=9000/mm^3
- Random blood glucose=310 mg/dL
- Urine glucose=Negative
- X-ray of the right foot=Negative

SYSTEMS REVIEW

◆ Cardiovascular/pulmonary
- BP: 145/80 mmHg
- Edema: None
- HR: 80 bpm
- RR: 13 bpm

◆ Integumentary

- Presence of scar formation: Noted at right great toe amputation site
- Skin color: WNL except wound perimeter that consists of thick, macerated callus
- Skin integrity: Open wound plantar surface of right great toe
♦ Musculoskeletal
  - Gross range of motion: WNL except limited ankle dorsiflexion and great toe extension
  - Gross strength: WNL
  - Gross symmetry: Feet asymmetrical due to prior amputation of the distal phalanx of the right great toe
  - Height: 6'0" (1.829 m)
  - Weight: 192 lbs (87.009 kg)
♦ Neuromuscular
  - Balance, gait, locomotion: Not impaired
  - Transfers, transitions: Not impaired
♦ Communication, affect, cognition, language, and learning style
  - Communication, affect, cognition: WNL
  - Learning preferences: Patient learns best by reading

TESTS AND MEASURES

♦ Anthropometric characteristics
  - BMI=26
  - Normal BMI ranges from 18.5 to 24.9
  - A BMI of 26 is defined as overweight[37]
♦ Assistive and adaptive devices: Ms. Donovan is not currently using any assistive devices
♦ Circulation
  - Pulse exam[38-40] (see Table 3-4)
    - Performed as an indicator of arterial blood flow
    - DP pulses B=3+, PT artery pulses B=2+
  - Capillary refill[41-47] (see Table 3-5)
    - Performed as an indicator of superficial blood flow
    - Capillary refill was 3 seconds both LEs
  - ABI[45,47-57] (see Table 3-6)
    - Performed because posterior tibial artery pulses were found to be diminished suggesting arterial insufficiency
    - The ABI will help determine the presence and severity of arterial insufficiency and assist with determining the plan of care
    - ABI was 1.0
♦ Cranial and peripheral nerve integrity
  - Protective sensation: Semmes-Weinstein monofilament testing[18-20,58,59] (Table 4-5)
    - Patients who are unable to sense the 5.07 monofilament (10 grams of pressure) on the plantar

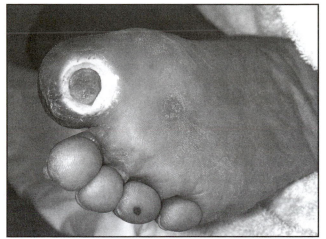

Figure 4-2. Full-thickness neuropathic wound right great toe. (See this figure in the Color Atlas following page 39.)

aspect of the foot have a loss of protective sensation and should be considered at risk for ulceration or reinjury due to insensitivity
    - Patient was unable to sense the 5.07 monofilament on either foot or ankle. She can detect the 5.07 monofilament proximal to her malleoli
♦ Gait, locomotion, and balance
  - Transfers: Unimpaired
  - Ambulates independently without significant deviation
  - Footwear: Old tennis-type shoes with significant wear pattern evident along lateral heel and medial forefoot
♦ Integumentary integrity
  - Associated skin
    - Skin color: WNL
    - Hair growth: WNL BLE
    - Nail growth: Slightly thickened, without discoloration
    - Temperature: Toes are warm to palpation
    - Texture/turgor: Skin appears anhydrous and cracked
    - Edema: Absent
  - Wound
    - Circular open wound noted on plantar aspect of the proximal phalanx of the right great toe
    - Full-thickness wound measures 3.2 x 2.8 cm, with a depth of 0.6 cm
    - Wound bed contains 100% pale granulation tissue
    - Wound drainage: Minimal, serosanguinous
    - Periwound contains thick, macerated callus

Table 4-5
SEMMES-WEINSTEIN MONOFILAMENT TESTING

Purpose	To identify the presence of protective sensation
Method	With the patient's vision occluded, apply the 5.07 monofilament perpendicular to the patient's skin surface with enough force to bend the filament
	Have the patient indicate when and where he/she perceives the filament is touching
	Randomly test each key landmark three times
	Plantar metatarsal heads 1, 3, and 5
	Plantar medial and lateral midfoot
	Plantar calcaneus
	Dorsal midfoot
	If the patient is unable to sense any of these landmarks, it may be prudent to continue testing more proximally to determine the most distal location that the patient is able to detect the monofilament
Interpretation	Able to detect 5.07 monofilament=Protective sensation
	Unable to detect 5.07 monofilament=Loss of protective sensation
Advantages	Quick, noninvasive, painless
	Reliable and valid test for the assessment of protective sensation in the foot
Limitations	Not accurate over areas of thick callus

- Signs of infection: None
- Activities, positions, and postures that produce or relieve trauma to the skin
  - Ms. Donovan wears an old tennis-type shoe without pressure relief and does not use an assistive device
- Muscle performance
  - Manual muscle testing revealed the following impairments: Foot intrinsics bilaterally=1+/5
- Pain
  - Patient denies toe/foot pain
- Range of motion
  - Ankle dorsiflexion=R 0 to 0 degrees, L 0 to 5 degrees
  - Gastrocnemius length=R lacks 8 degrees from neutral, L 0 to 0 degrees
  - Great toe extension=R 0 to 45 degrees, L 0 to 58 degrees
- Self-care and home management
  - Self-care
    - During the interview Ms. Donovan reports she has some difficulty positioning her leg so she can check the bottom of her foot to see the wound
    - She reports she usually tries to eat a balanced diet but does not always have the time to do so
    - She reports having difficulty avoiding desserts
  - Home management
    - Ms. Donovan walks within her house, to and from the bus stop, and does her own shopping and errands in old tennis-type shoes without pressure relief and without an assistive device

- Work, community, and leisure integration or reintegration
  - Ms. Donovan walks occasionally at work

EVALUATION

Ms. Donovan's history and risk factors previously outlined indicate that she is an overweight smoker and a non-exerciser with poorly controlled Type 2 diabetes and peripheral vascular disease. She has a family history of cardiovascular disease and obesity. She has had a previous nonhealing ulcer that required amputation and a worsening, full-thickness wound due to neuropathy that would be classified as a Wagner Grade I ulcer (see Pattern B: Impaired Integumentary Integrity Associated With Superficial Skin Involvement for ulcer classification). She has decreased ankle and great toe ROM, muscle performance, and protective sensation and limitations in self-care.

DIAGNOSIS

Ms. Donovan has a neuropathic wound with full-thickness skin involvement and scar formation. She has impaired: circulation; cranial and peripheral nerve integrity; integumentary integrity; muscle performance; and range of motion. She is functionally limited in self-care and home management actions, tasks, and activities. These findings are consistent with placement in Pattern D: Impaired Integumentary Integrity Associated With Full-Thickness Skin Involvement and Scar Formation. These impairments and functional limitations will be addressed in determining the prognosis and the plan of care.

PROGNOSIS AND PLAN OF CARE

Over the course of the visits, the following mutually established outcomes have been determined:

♦ Ability to perform physical activities related to self-care and work is improved

♦ Knowledge of behaviors that foster healthy habits, wellness, and prevention is increased

♦ Patient/family knowledge and awareness of diagnosis, prognosis, interventions, and anticipated goals and outcomes are increased

♦ Physical function is improved

♦ Referrals are made to other professionals or resources

♦ Risk factors are reduced

♦ Risk of recurrence is reduced

♦ Risk of secondary impairment is reduced

♦ ROM is improved

♦ Skin integrity is restored

♦ Tissue perfusion and oxygenation are enhanced

To achieve these outcomes, the appropriate interventions for this patient are determined. These will include: coordination, communication, and documentation; patient/client-related instruction; therapeutic exercise; functional training in self-care and home management; functional training in work, community, and leisure integration or reintegration; prescription, application, and, as appropriate, fabrication of devices and equipment; integumentary repair and protection techniques; and physical agents and mechanical modalities.

Based on the diagnosis and prognosis, Ms. Donovan is expected to require between 10 to 16 visits over a 4-week period of time. Ms. Donovan lives alone, is motivated, and is trying to adhere to her home program. She is not severely impaired and is fairly healthy.

INTERVENTIONS

RATIONALE FOR SELECTED INTERVENTIONS

Therapeutic Exercise

Exercise is extremely important for this patient since impairments in ankle dorsiflexion and great toe extension are believed to play a role in the development and progression of neuropathic ulcerations by increasing plantar pressure and shear forces.[1,12,17,21,60-62] Gains in flexibility may be maximized by performing three stretches of 30-second duration.[63]

Intrinsic foot muscle weakness, likely due to autonomic neuropathy, may predispose patients with diabetes to neuropathic ulceration by increasing plantar pressure and shear forces.[22,23] Therefore, strengthening exercises will be incorporated into her program.

Aerobic exercise may assist with weight loss and improved glycemic control.[2,37] A fairly light intensity (30% to 49% of target HR) was chosen as a starting point because this patient has been sedentary and a non-exerciser. The ultimate goal of exercising at a somewhat hard intensity (50% to 74% of target HR) was set because this is the intensity suggested for the average patient.[64]

Gait and locomotion training will also be incorporated into her program. Off-loading of neuropathic ulcerations decreases pressure and shear forces on the wound to allow healing to occur.[16] Because she is overweight, sedentary, and has neuropathic changes, it was considered unlikely that Ms. Donovan would be able or willing to ambulate using a nonweightbearing pattern. Therefore, partial weightbearing with crutches or a walker was chosen. A step-to pattern and smaller steps has been shown to decrease forefoot plantar pressures and shear forces.[65,66]

Prescription, Application, and, as Appropriate, Fabrication of Devices and Equipment

A walking shoe should be selected for this patient for the following reasons.[1,16,27] A rocker-bottom will decrease forefoot pressure or shear forces. The walking shoe can be modified with a pressure-reducing insole to further decrease pressure over the patient's first ray during standing and walking. Since the shoe has enclosed toes, it will decrease the risk of foreign objects entering the shoe. It also allows room for her wound dressings. Compared to a padded ankle-foot orthosis, the walking shoe is less bulky, lighter, more stable, and provides ease of walking. Compared to a total contact cast, the walking shoe is less restrictive and allows for daily wound inspection, wound management, and therapeutic exercise. With appropriate insole and dressing, the walking shoe will likely be as effective as the total contact cast in reducing pressure and shear forces at the plantar aspect of the first proximal phalanx.

Integumentary Repair and Protection Techniques

Integumentary repair and protection techniques will be important for this patient. All areas of the wound bed should be thoroughly probed to ensure there are no tunnels, undermined areas, or exposed deep tissues. Sharp debridement of callus is indicated, because calluses produce localized areas of increased plantar pressure.[1,67] Keratinocytes will build up on the edge of the wound in the presence of callus rather than growing across the wound bed.

A petrolatum-based moisturizer will be applied to Ms. Donovan's intact skin to help improve skin pliability and minimize dry, cracked, and callused skin that results from autonomic neuropathy. The moisturizer should not be applied between the toes or on the wound. A skin sealant applied to the periwound will help decrease maceration from wound drainage.[27]

Moisture-retentive dressings are used to enhance wound healing in several ways. They maintain a moist, warm wound environment and are associated with lower rates of wound infection. They do not traumatize the wound bed upon removal. Specifically, a sheet of hydrogel has the following advantages: it provides cushioning to decrease the adverse effects of pressure; it is minimally adhesive and, therefore, will not traumatize fragile skin upon removal; and it is appropriate for wounds with minimal drainage.[27,68-71]

Physical Agents and Mechanical Modalities

In this case, wound irrigation with normal saline is the treatment of choice since it removes loosely adhered debris, bacteria, dressing residue, and old topical agents. It may decrease the risk of infection and promotes moist wound healing. Irrigation with saline is less expensive than pulsatile lavage with suction.[72-74]

Because of the acuity of Ms. Donovan's wound and lack of unloading of the involved area, it was decided that more aggressive wound management interventions, such as electrical stimulation or pulsatile lavage with suction, were not warranted at this time. Should the wound fail to improve in a timely manner, these interventions will be reconsidered.

COORDINATION, COMMUNICATION, AND DOCUMENTATION

Ms. Donovan's family will be encouraged to be actively involved to provide support for her as she tries to modify her diet and lifestyle. Her primary care physician will be contacted regarding her elevated blood glucose levels to assist with pharmacological modifications as needed. The clinician will request a referral to an orthotist to provide permanent footwear to decrease the risk of ulceration of her uninvolved foot and to decrease the risk of recurrence after the present ulcer has healed.[1,75,76] Her primary care physician will also be notified if she thinks that she may benefit from pharmacological interventions to assist her with smoking cessation. A consult with a diabetic educator will be requested to assist Ms. Donovan with following an appropriate diet to better manage her diabetes. All elements of the patient's management will be documented.

PATIENT/CLIENT-RELATED INSTRUCTION

Ms. Donovan will be instructed in the risk factors for neuropathic ulcers, wound infection, and amputation. Particular emphasis will be placed on:

♦ Maintaining near normal blood sugar control that will facilitate wound healing and decrease the development and progression of the long-term complications of dia-

betes, such as retinopathy, nephropathy, and neuropathy[28,29]

♦ Optimizing glycemic control by[28,29,77]:
  ● Performing regular aerobic exercise to facilitate improved blood sugar control and weight loss
  ● Following a diet provided by the patient's dietician that is low in fat and simple sugars to also facilitate improved blood sugar control and weight loss
  ● Adjusting food intake and hypoglycemic agent dosage based on the result of frequent daily blood sugar monitoring

♦ Stopping smoking since smoking delays wound healing by causing vasoconstriction, increased platelet aggregation, and reduced oxygen availability[35,78]

♦ Understanding of the fact that her wound is caused by the neuropathy that results in a lack of protective sensation or lack of an early warning signal for tissue damage; therefore, pain, or the lack thereof, is not an adequate indicator of tissue trauma

♦ Avoiding skin trauma by[12]:
  ● Protecting against excessive heat or cold (bath water, heating pads, and environmental)
  ● Not using chemicals, such as corn removers, unless directed to do so by a clinician
  ● Using a mirror to assist with daily skin inspection of all surfaces of both feet and ankles for signs of trauma, irritation, or excessive pressure
  ● Always wearing footwear to decrease the risk of minor skin trauma, such as stepping on a sharp object[12,19]
    ■ Shoes should fit properly, be comfortable, easy to don/doff, and have enclosed toes
    ■ Inspect soles and insides of shoes visually and with a hand for foreign objects before donning
    ■ Always wear socks with shoes, preferably white socks without seams or tight elastic cuffs, to allow easy visualization of overt skin trauma and to prevent edema[27]
    ■ Break in new shoes slowly
    ■ In cold weather, wear insulated boots or ensure shoes provide sufficient room for heavy socks

♦ Understanding of the facts that open wounds or inappropriately bandaged wounds provide a direct pathway for bacteria to enter the body, increasing the risk of infection, osteomyelitis, and amputation

♦ Instructing the patient in the signs and symptoms of infection and action plan if these occur

♦ Instructing the patient in proper wound management

♦ Providing her with written copies of all instructional materials, HEP, and self-care techniques because her preferred learning style is review of written information

THERAPEUTIC EXERCISE

- ♦ Aerobic capacity/endurance conditioning
  - • Parameters
    - ■ Mode: Upper body ergometer or stationary bicycle avoiding right forefoot pressure
    - ■ Intensity: Borg rate of perceived exertion (Table 4-6)[79] 11 (fairly light) to 13 (somewhat hard)
    - ■ Duration: Gradually increase as tolerated until able to perform continuously for 20 to 30 minutes
    - ■ Frequency: Ideally 5 to 7 days per week
  - • Precautions
    - ■ Monitor blood sugar response to increased activity
    - ■ Have fast-acting carbohydrate nearby in the event of a hypolgycemic reaction
    - ■ Do not exercise during peak action time of hypoglycemic agents
- ♦ Flexibility exercises
  - • Stretching exercises should be done after warming up, using a slow and steady stretch accompanied by deep breathing, and building hold up to 30 seconds
  - • Gastrocnemius stretching: Sitting in a chair, extend knee, use a bathrobe tie looped around the ball of the foot to assist with ankle dorsiflexion
  - • Dorsiflexion stretching: Repeat above stretch with knee flexed approximately 90 degrees
  - • Great toe extension: With bandage on, grasp sides of right great toe and gently stretch into extension
  - • Perform bilaterally for three repetitions each once daily
- ♦ Gait and locomotion training
  - • Instruct patient in partial weightbearing with crutches or walker
  - • Take smaller steps and use a step-to pattern
- ♦ Strength, power, and endurance training
  - • Perform bilaterally for 1 minute, two to three times daily
    - ■ Ankle pumps
    - ■ Toe wiggling/AROM

FUNCTIONAL TRAINING IN SELF-CARE AND HOME MANAGEMENT

- ♦ Self-care
  - • Monitor blood sugar at least daily to assist with improved glycemic control
  - • Twice daily skin inspection of all surfaces of both feet and ankles for signs of trauma, irritation, or excessive pressure
  - • Optimize nutrition by following through with dietician recommendations

Table 4-6

RATE OF PERCEIVED EXERTION SCALE

Numerical Scale	Verbal Descriptor	% Heart Rate Max Reserve
6		
7	Very, very light	
8		
9	Very light	<30
10		
11	Fairly light	30 to 49
12		
13	Somewhat hard	50 to 74
14		
15	Hard	75 to 84
16		
17	Very hard	>85
18		
19	Very, very hard	
20		

- ■ Weekly meal planning to improve nutritional quality
- ■ Buying snacks and desserts that are appealing, convenient, and healthy
- ■ Perusing the local bookstore's cookbook selections to find new, appealing, and healthy meal choices
- ♦ Home management
  - • Limit her walking distance and time for home management activities as much as possible
    - ■ Request assistance from family/friends for rides to the store to decrease walking distance
    - ■ Avoid unnecessary errands
    - ■ Plan ahead to decrease the amount of required walking

FUNCTIONAL TRAINING IN WORK, COMMUNITY, AND LEISURE INTEGRATION OR REINTEGRATION

- ♦ Work
  - • Bring a nutritious lunch and snack to work to decrease the need for buying fast food or snacks high in fat or sugar
  - • Request assistance from family/friends for rides to work to decrease walking distance to and from the bus stop
- ♦ Leisure
  - • Consider joining a health club to assist with weight loss and improved glycemic control
  - • To help make exercise fun and a daily routine, encourage family members to join as well

PRESCRIPTION, APPLICATION, AND, AS APPROPRIATE, FABRICATION OF DEVICES AND EQUIPMENT

♦ Ms. Donovan will be fitted with an appropriately sized walking shoe with a rocker-bottom, enclosed toe, and pressure-reducing insole with relief at, and distal to, the first MTP

INTEGUMENTARY REPAIR AND PROTECTION TECHNIQUES

♦ Dressings
  ● The periwound skin will be covered with the primary dressing
  ● A sheet of hydrogel will be applied to the patient's wound and secured with a bulky gauze dressing
♦ Topical agents
  ● Twice daily, a nonperfumed, low pH moisturizer will be applied to her lower legs and feet, except between her toes and on the periwound skin
  ● A skin sealant will be applied to the areas of periwound skin

PHYSICAL AGENTS AND MECHANICAL MODALITIES

♦ Hydrotherapy
  ● The wound will be irrigated with normal saline using a 35-mL syringe and a 19-gauge angiocatheter

ANTICIPATED GOALS AND EXPECTED OUTCOMES

♦ Impact on pathology/pathophysiology
  ● No cracks in right plantar skin surface are identifiable in 2 weeks.
  ● Periwound maceration and callus are resolved in 2 weeks.
  ● Tissue perfusion and oxygenation are enhanced.
  ● Wound bed shows evidence of epithelialization at all borders in 1 week.
♦ Impact on impairments
  ● Integumentary integrity is restored in 4 weeks.
  ● Right first MTP extension measures 0 to 60 degrees in 3 weeks.
  ● Right gastrocnemius length measures 0 to 5 degrees in 3 weeks.
♦ Impact on functional limitations
  ● Patient is able to walk in appropriate footwear without a decline in skin status in 4 weeks.
  ● Patient is independently walking with step-to pattern

using bilateral crutches or a walker and walking shoe in two visits.
♦ Risk reduction/prevention
  ● Risk factors are reduced.
  ● Risk of recurrence is reduced.
  ● Self-management of symptoms is improved.
♦ Impact on health, wellness, and fitness
  ● Fitness is improved.
  ● Health status is improved.
  ● Physical function is improved.
♦ Impact on societal resources
  ● A referral is made to a certified diabetic educator to assist patient with glycemic control in 1 week.
  ● A referral is made to the patient's primary care physician to address inadequate glycemic control and smoking cessation programs in 1 week.
  ● Resources are utilized in a cost-effective way.
  ● Utilization of physical therapy services is optimized.
♦ Patient/client satisfaction
  ● Care is coordinated with patient and other health care professionals.
  ● Documentation occurs throughout patient management and follows APTA's *Guidelines for Physical Therapy Documentation*.[80]
  ● Patient knowledge and awareness of the diagnosis, prognosis, interventions, and anticipated goals and outcomes are increased.
  ● Patient understanding of anticipated goals and expected outcomes is increased.

REEXAMINATION

Reexamination is performed throughout the episode of care.

DISCHARGE

Ms. Donovan is discharged from physical therapy after a total of 12 physical therapy sessions and attainment of her goals and expectations. These sessions have covered her entire episode of care. She is discharged because she has achieved her anticipated goals and expected outcomes.

PSYCHOLOGICAL ASPECTS

To maximize compliance and outcomes, Ms. Donovan will be encouraged to involve her family in all aspects of her care. Because her previous neuropathic ulceration resulted in amputation, the physical therapist must highlight the control she has over the current situation and that, by adhering to the preceding plan of care, wound healing is possible.

Realistic goal setting, such as a time frame for smoking cessation, a goal of eating only one high sugar/high fat dessert per week, or exercising aerobically every other day for the first 2 weeks, may be beneficial in helping her make necessary lifestyle changes.

Case Study #2:
Full-Thickness Traumatic and Arterial Insufficiency Wound

Mrs. Bridget Carter is a 69-year-old female who has a wound on her right anterior lower leg (Figure 4-3).

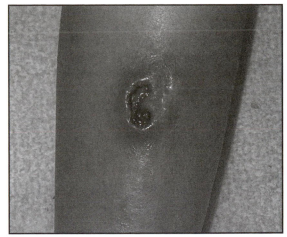

Figure 4-3. Full-thickness traumatic and arterial insufficiency wound right anterior lower leg. (See this figure in the Color Atlas following page 39.)

PHYSICAL THERAPIST EXAMINATION

HISTORY

- General demographics: Mrs. Carter is a 69-year-old female whose primary language is English. She is right-hand dominant and has an associate's degree.
- Social history: She is widowed and has two sons and one granddaughter who live in the same town.
- Employment/work: Mrs. Carter worked as a licensed practical nurse (LPN) at a local home health agency until she retired 6 years ago.
- Living environment: She lives alone in a one-story house with two steps to enter with a railing.
- General health status
  - General health perception: Mrs. Carter reports that her health status is fair.
  - Physical function: She reports her physical function is limited due to poor balance.
  - Psychological function: Normal.
  - Role function: Mother, grandmother.
  - Social function: Mrs. Carter is active in the local women's auxiliary.
- Social/health habits: She is a nondrinker and quit smoking approximately 20 years ago.
- Family history: She reports both parents died in an auto accident before the age of 40, her grandparents lived into their 80s and died of natural causes.
- Medical/surgical history: Mrs. Carter has Type 2 diabetes mellitus, cataracts, HTN, peripheral neuropathy, OA, and had a myocardial infarction 2 years ago. She reports her blood sugars are generally 90 to 120 mg/dL. She reports no history of falls.
- Current condition(s)/chief complaint(s): She complains of a painful hematoma that began about a month ago when she hit her shin on the coffee table in her living room. She reports the bruise was initially nearly twice as raised as it is currently and never drained. She became concerned when the skin turned black and there was an increase in redness around the wound. She has not had any treatment for the hematoma.
- Functional status and activity level: Mrs. Carter reports limitations in IADL due to decreased balance and fatigue. She is unable to drive due to her cataracts. She is a non-exerciser.
- Medications: Insulin, warfarin, propranolol, Neurontin, naproxen

SYSTEMS REVIEW

- Cardiovascular/pulmonary
  - BP: 175/84 mmHg
  - Edema: Slight bilateral ankles
  - HR: 64 bpm
  - RR: 14 bpm
- Integumentary
  - Presence of scar formation: None
  - Skin color: Periwound erythema
  - Skin integrity: Open wound right anterior lower leg
- Musculoskeletal
  - Gross range of motion: BLE WNL for patient's age
  - Gross strength: BLE grossly 4/5
  - Gross symmetry: Symmetrical
  - Height: 5'10" (1.78 m)
  - Weight: 188 lbs (85.28 kg)
- Neuromuscular
  - Transfers require UE assist

- Gait is unsteady without assistive device
♦ Communication, affect, cognition, language, and learning style
  - Communication, affect, cognition: WNL
  - Learning preferences: Patient learns best by listening

TESTS AND MEASURES

♦ Anthropometric characteristics
  - BMI=27
  - Normal BMI ranges from 18.5 to 24.9
  - A BMI of 27 is defined as overweight[37]
♦ Assistive and adaptive devices
  - Patient uses a small-based quad cane
♦ Circulation
  - Pulse exam[38-40] (see Table 3-4)
    - Performed as an indicator of arterial blood flow
    - Bilateral popliteal pulses 2+
    - Bilateral DP and PT arteries 1+
  - Capillary refill[41-47] (see Table 3-5)
    - Performed as an indicator of superficial blood flow
    - Capillary refill bilaterally 5 seconds
  - ABI[45,47-57] (see Table 3-6)
    - Performed because her history indicates a risk of peripheral vascular disease and pedal pulses were diminished, suggesting arterial insufficiency
    - The ABI will help determine the severity of arterial insufficiency and assist with determining the plan of care
    - ABI=0.7 R and 0.8 L
  - Homans' sign[81-84] (see Table 3-8)
    - Performed as a screening procedure on patients with suspected peripheral vascular disease to identify the presence of a DVT because of the potentially devastating consequences of a DVT (eg, pulmonary embolism)
    - Negative bilaterally
    - Alternative: Because of the potentially devastating consequences of a DVT (eg, pulmonary embolism) and the poor reliability of the Homans' sign, the reader is referred to the scoring system developed by Anand for an alternate screening strategy that more accurately predicts the presence of a DVT[84,85]
♦ Cranial and peripheral nerve integrity
  - Semmes-Weinstein monofilament testing[18-20,58,59]
    - Performed due to her history of diabetes
    - Patients who are unable to sense the 5.07 monofilament (10 g of pressure) on the plantar aspect of the foot have a loss of protective sensation and should be considered at risk for ulceration or reinjury due to insensitivity

- She is unable to detect 5.07 monofilament distal to the proximal tibia bilaterally
♦ Gait, locomotion, and balance
  - Transfers require use of UEs
  - Ambulation
    - Reports fatigue after walking 200 feet, mildly unsteady which increases with increase in distance
    - During ambulation, vital signs increased
      ‣ HR to 80 bpm
      ‣ BP to 180/84 mmHg
      ‣ RR to 20 bpm
  - Modified Gait Abnormality Rating Scale (GARS-M)[86-88]
    - Since Mrs. Carter has an unsteady gait and peripheral neuropathy, this test was performed to better quantify her gait deviations and to assess for fall risk
    - The GARS-M is a simple clinical assessment of gait deviations developed to assess fall risk in community dwelling individuals
    - Patient scores range from 0 to 3 on seven items including variability, path deviation, and ROM
    - Higher scores indicate greater risk of falling
    - Scores over 8 indicate a risk of falls
    - Score: 8
  - Berg Balance test[86,89-91]
    - Since she has an unsteady gait and peripheral neuropathy, this test was performed to determine her fall risk
    - The Berg Balance test is a simple clinical balance assessment that rates 14 static and dynamic functional tests such as sitting, rising, and tandem stance on a 0 to 4 scale
    - Lower scores indicate greater fall risk
    - Score less than 45 is predictive of multiple falls
    - Score: 40/56
♦ Integumentary integrity
  - Associated skin
    - Skin color: Erythema extending 2.2 cm laterally and superiorly, 0.4 cm medially from wound margin
    - Hair growth: Absent lower legs
    - Nail growth: Normal
    - Temperature: Toes are slightly cool to palpation
    - Texture/turgor: Skin appears thin and fragile
    - Edema: 1+ edema dorsal feet and ankles, calf circumferential measurements symmetrical
  - Activities, positioning, and postures that produce or relieve trauma to the skin
    - Potential for skin damage due to trauma (secondary to poor vision, instability, and neuropathy)

- Wound
  - Irregular-shaped, open wound right anterior lower leg
  - Wound is raised approximately 1 cm above the surrounding skin surface
  - Wound measures 2.1 cm in length, superior width 1.0 cm, inferior width 1.1 cm, depth unable to be determined prior to debridement
  - Wound bed consists of 100% eschar
  - Wound drainage: None
  - After sharp debridement of eschar and significant amounts of gelatinous, clotted blood, the following was determined:
  - Full-thickness wound with a depth of 0.6 cm
  - 70% granular, 20% adherent slough and coagulated blood inferiorly, 10% fat/fascia at 3 o'clock position within undermined area
  - Undermining present from 1 o'clock to 6 o'clock, with a maximum of 2.1 cm at 3 o'clock
  - The wound was flush with surrounding tissue and there was a decrease in periwound erythema (see Figure 4-3)
- Muscle performance: Unimpaired when assessed by way of manual muscle testing
- Pain
  - Mrs. Carter rates her wound pain as a 3/10 on the VAS[92-94]
- Range of motion: Unimpaired
- Self-care and home management
  - During the interview Mrs. Carter reported that her poor vision prohibited skin checks or reading anything other than large print, including a glucometer
  - She has a home health aide assist with medications, bathing, and housework
  - Mrs. Carter generally walks without an assistive device in her home despite feeling unsteady
  - She occasionally uses a small-based quad cane to ambulate outside of the home
  - She reports she is unable to walk through the grocery store secondary to fatigue
- Work, community, and leisure integration or reintegration
  - Leisure
    - Twice a week a friend brings Mrs. Carter to meetings of the women's auxiliary

EVALUATION

Mrs. Carter's history and risk factors previously outlined indicate that she is a sedentary female with cardiovascular, peripheral vascular, eye, and kidney disease. She has a non-healing, full-thickness wound due to the combined effects of trauma and arterial insufficiency. Mrs. Carter lacks protective sensation in her feet. She has decreased balance and mobility and is at risk for falls. She has limitations in self-care.

DIAGNOSIS

Mrs. Carter has a traumatic and arterial insufficiency wound with full-thickness skin involvement and scar formation and has wound pain. She has impaired: anthropometric characteristics; circulation; cranial and peripheral nerve integrity; gait, locomotion, and balance; and integumentary integrity. She is functionally limited in self-care and home management and in work, community, and leisure actions, tasks, and activities. These findings are consistent with placement in Pattern D: Impaired Integumentary Integrity Associated With Full-Thickness Skin Involvement and Scar Formation. These impairments and functional limitations will be addressed in determining the prognosis and the plan of care.

PROGNOSIS AND PLAN OF CARE

Over the course of the visits, the following mutually established outcomes have been determined:
- Gait, locomotion, and balance are improved
- Knowledge of behaviors that foster healthy habits, wellness, and prevention is increased
- Patient/family knowledge and awareness of diagnosis, prognosis, interventions, and anticipated goals and outcomes are increased
- Physical function is improved
- Risk factors are reduced
- Risk of recurrence is reduced
- Risk of secondary impairment is reduced
- Skin integrity is restored
- Tissue perfusion and oxygenation are enhanced

To achieve these outcomes, the appropriate interventions for this patient are determined. These will include: coordination, communication, and documentation; patient/client-related instruction; therapeutic exercise; functional training in self-care and home management; functional training in work, community, and leisure integration or reintegration; integumentary repair and protection techniques; and physical agents and mechanical modalities.

Based on the diagnosis and prognosis, Mrs. Carter is expected to require between three to five visits over a 3-week period of time. Mrs. Carter lives alone but has assistance available for wound and skin care. Although she has impaired circulation, she has sufficient blood flow to support wound healing. Mrs. Carter has impaired sensation, vision, and mobility, placing her at risk for further injury and skin breakdown. However, she is motivated and has a good understanding of wound etiology and self-management techniques from her previous job as an LPN.

INTERVENTIONS

RATIONALE FOR SELECTED INTERVENTIONS

Therapeutic Exercise

Since the results of her testing using the GARS-M and Berg Balance test scores[86-91] indicated that she is at risk for falls, therapeutic exercises will be incorporated into her program. The Berg Balance test revealed deficits in dynamic balance and when a narrow base of support was required. Therefore, balance activities will stress these two areas.

An assistive device will increase her base of support, and specific gait training will improve her dynamic balance. Therapeutic exercises have been shown to improve balance, postural stability, and functional mobility and to decrease the risk of falls.[95-99]

Aerobic capacity/endurance training exercises can assist with weight loss, improved glycemic control, and walking endurance.[2] A fairly light intensity (11 to 12 on the Borg Rate of Perceived Exertion Scale) was chosen because Mrs. Carter is a sedentary, non-exerciser with multiple medical problems. maximum HR response will not be accurate with her due to the use of beta-blockers.[64]

Integumentary Repair and Protection Techniques

Sharp debridement will be used with this patient since it decreases the risk of infection by reducing bacterial concentration within the wound bed and improving the bactericidal activity of leukocytes. It shortens the inflammatory phase of wound healing and decreases the energy required for wound healing. Sharp debridement eliminates a physical barrier to wound healing by removing dead tissue and debris.[100-102]

A skin sealant applied to the periwound will help decrease maceration from wound drainage. Moisture-retentive dressings will also be used to enhance wound healing. They maintain a moist, warm wound environment and are associated with lower rates of wound infection. They absorb sufficient wound drainage to allow decreased dressing frequency and encourage autolytic debridement of remaining slough. Moisture-retentive dressings are associated with lower costs than traditional gauze bandages. They decrease patient pain complaint and do not traumatize the wound bed upon removal. They are easier to apply and will not obstruct blood flow like a gauze wrap may. Specifically, a hydrocolloid enhances wound healing by providing a thermal insulation, absorbing wound drainage, and staying in place for several days.[27,68,69,71,103,104]

A moisturizer applied to her intact skin will help improve skin pliability and decrease the risk of future skin damage from minor trauma or irritation.[27]

Physical Agents and Mechanical Modalities

For this patient wound irrigation will be done with normal saline since it removes loosely adhered debris, bacteria, dressing residue, and old topical agents. It may decrease the risk of infection and promotes moist wound healing. Pulsatile lavage with suction is not appropriate for her at this time due to the presence of gelatinous coagulated blood and ongoing use of a blood thinning agent. In addition, whirlpool is not appropriate for her at this time due to the need for dependent positioning that would exacerbate her edema.[72-74,105,106]

COORDINATION, COMMUNICATION, AND DOCUMENTATION

Care will be coordinated with her home health aide. Mrs. Carter's primary care physician will be contacted regarding her BP and symmetrical bilateral LE edema. All elements of the patient's management will be documented.

PATIENT/CLIENT-RELATED INSTRUCTION

Mrs. Carter will be instructed in the risk factors for traumatic and vascular insufficiency ulcers. Particular emphasis will be placed on:

♦ Understanding that open wounds or inappropriately bandaged wounds provide a direct pathway for bacteria to enter the body, increasing the risk of infection and sepsis
♦ Instructing the patient and home health aide in the signs and symptoms of infection and action plan if these occur
♦ Instructing the patient and home health aide in proper wound management
♦ Understanding that arterial insufficiency limits blood flow, proper nutrition, and oxygenation to affected areas
♦ Optimizing her blood flow by:
  • Avoiding constrictive clothing such as tight elastic socks or elastic pant leg cuffs
  • Avoiding excessive leg elevation
♦ Avoiding skin trauma by:
  • Being aware of potential obstacles, such as table edges that, if bumped against, may traumatize fragile skin
  • Protecting against excessive heat or cold (bath water, heating pads, and environmental)
  • Not using chemicals, such as corn removers, unless directed to do so by a clinician
  • Having her home health aide inspect her skin for signs of trauma, irritation, or excessive pressure
♦ Presenting her with patient information and education materials orally until she is able to verbalize understand-

ing of the material addressed, since she learns best by listening and has poor visual acuity

♦ Providing her with written copies of instructional materials, HEP, and self-care techniques to improve follow through with her home health aide

THERAPEUTIC EXERCISE

♦ Aerobic capacity/endurance conditioning
  • Gradually progress walking time until able to walk for 15 minutes uninterrupted without fatigue
  • Stationary bicycle
    ▪ Intensity
      ‣ Teach Mrs. Carter how to use the Borg Rate of Perceived Exertion scale
      ‣ Strive to maintain exercise intensity of approximately 11 (fairly light)
    ▪ Duration
      ‣ Beginning with interrupted cycling for 5 minutes
      ‣ Increase cycle time and decrease rest time until able to cycle 5 minutes uninterrupted
      ‣ Gradually increase cycling time until able to cycle uninterrupted for 15 to 20 minutes
    ▪ Frequency
      ‣ 4 to 6 days per week
♦ Balance, coordination, and agility training
  • Dynamic weight shifts
  • Balancing on toes/heels
  • Standing with eyes open/closed while moving UEs
  • Side stepping and braiding
  • Performed one to two times per day
♦ Gait and locomotion training
  • She will be instructed in the use of a small-based quad cane
  • Practice ambulating using the cane and appropriate gait pattern in the house several times per day

FUNCTIONAL TRAINING IN SELF-CARE AND HOME MANAGEMENT

♦ Self-care
  • Because of her lack of protective sensation and poor visual acuity, her home health aide will be shown how to perform daily skin checks on her to identify early signs of the adverse effects of pressure or trauma
♦ Home management
  • Mrs. Carter will be asked to perform a home safety check to minimize fall risks
  • Avoiding potential fall hazards may include attention to the following:
    ▪ The presence of rails at the front entry steps
    ▪ Appropriate lighting
      ‣ Outside lights to illuminate the front walkway where she is dropped off and at the front steps and stoop
      ‣ A light or motion sensor may be helpful
      ‣ Turning the lights on before moving from room to room in the evening
      ‣ Leaving a bathroom light on at night to illuminate potential obstacles
    ▪ Floors
      ‣ Throw rugs should be either eliminated or secured to prevent slippage
      ‣ Mrs. Carter should be wary at the transition between rooms and between surfaces (wood, tile, and carpeted flooring) to prevent tripping on uneven or irregular surfaces
      ‣ Floors should be kept free of clutter
    ▪ Bathroom
      ‣ Rails in shower or tub, grab bar by the commode
      ‣ A bath bench and removable shower head may be indicated
      ‣ A non-skid bath mat to prevent slipping on the wet floor
    ▪ General home management
      ‣ Adequate room should be available to walk between furniture such as sofas, chairs, and coffee tables
      ‣ Extension and phone cords should be kept out of the line of foot traffic
      ‣ Spills should be cleaned up immediately

FUNCTIONAL TRAINING IN WORK, COMMUNITY, AND LEISURE INTEGRATION OR REINTEGRATION

♦ Leisure
  • Intermittent, short walks will be encouraged to assist with LE circulation and improving ambulatory and cardiovascular endurance
  • Mrs. Carter may want to consider purchasing a stationary bicycle to enhance cardiovascular fitness and assist with the management of HTN, glycemic control, weight management, and LE OA
  • Because of the benefits of increased activity and socialization, Mrs. Carter should be encouraged to continue her involvement with the women's auxiliary

INTEGUMENTARY REPAIR AND PROTECTION TECHNIQUES

♦ Debridement: Selective

- The thick, dry eschar initially present was selectively debrided with a scalpel
- Coagulated blood and slough were debrided as much as possible to reveal the wound bed described above
- The remaining slough will be debrided as needed/able with each dressing change
  ◆ Dressings
    - A sheet of hydrocolloid will be applied to her wound
    - The dressing will be signed, dated, and left in place for 5 days
    - If strike-through occurs, the dressing will be changed more often
  ◆ Topical agents
    - A skin sealant will be applied to the areas of periwound skin that will be covered with the primary dressing
    - A nonperfumed, low pH moisturizer will be applied once or twice daily to her lower legs and feet, except between her toes and on periwound skin

PHYSICAL AGENTS AND MECHANICAL MODALITIES

◆ The wound will be irrigated with normal saline using a 35-mL syringe with a 19-gauge angiocatheter

ANTICIPATED GOALS AND EXPECTED OUTCOMES

◆ Impact on pathology/pathophysiology
  - Debridement of nonviable tissue is achieved in 2 weeks.
  - Right lower leg pain is resolved in 3 weeks.
  - Tissue perfusion and oxygenation are enhanced.
◆ Impact on impairments
  - Aerobic capacity/endurance is increased and patient is able to walk 15 minutes and ride a bicycle 10 minutes in 3 weeks.
  - Circulation in the LE is increased.
  - Gait, locomotion, and balance are improved.
  - Integumentary integrity is restored in 3 weeks.
◆ Impact on functional limitations
  - Ability to perform physical actions, tasks, or activities related to self-care, home management, work, and leisure is improved.
  - Patient is able to walk 15 minutes with small-based quad cane without loss of balance or fatigue in 3 weeks.
  - Patient will have home environment modifications performed, such as removal of throw rugs, installation of bath mats and a bath chair or bench, and

removal of unnecessary clutter blocking traffic patterns, to decrease risk of falls or injury.
◆ Risk reduction/prevention
  - Behaviors that foster healthy habits, wellness, and prevention are acquired.
  - Patient and home health aide are independent with skin checks to identify areas of excessive pressure, shear, or skin breakdown in 1 week.
  - Risk factors are reduced.
  - Risk of recurrence is reduced.
  - Risk of secondary impairment is reduced.
  - Self-management of symptoms is improved.
◆ Impact on health, wellness, and fitness
  - Fitness is improved.
  - Health status is improved.
  - Physical function is improved.
◆ Impact on societal resources
  - Resources are utilized in a cost-effective way.
  - Utilization of physical therapy services is optimized.
◆ Patient/client satisfaction
  - Care is coordinated with patient and her home health aide.
  - Documentation occurs throughout patient management and follows APTA's *Guidelines for Physical Therapy Documentation.*[80]
  - Patient knowledge and awareness of the diagnosis, prognosis, interventions, and anticipated goals and outcomes are increased.
  - Patient understanding of anticipated goals and expected outcomes is increased.

REEXAMINATION

Reexamination is performed throughout the episode of care.

DISCHARGE

Mrs. Carter is discharged from physical therapy after a total of four physical therapy sessions and attainment of her goals and expectations. These sessions have covered her entire episode of care. She is discharged because she has achieved her anticipated goals and expected outcomes.

PSYCHOLOGICAL ASPECTS

Because of Mrs. Carter's previous experience as an LPN, information about wound pathophysiology and interventions may be provided at a more medically oriented level. In addition, the clinician should try to ascertain her previous professional experience with patients with similar medical conditions and relate her current situation to those of other patients she may have encountered in the past. While emphasizing her autonomy, she should be encouraged to draw upon the resources she has available (home health aide, family, and friends) to assist her in the portions of her care that require assistance, such as skin checks and wound management.

Case Study #3:
Full-Thickness Infected Wound

Mr. Steven Dawson is a 37-year-old male who has a nonhealing, infected wound on the dorsal aspect of his left foot and had undergone surgery for brain cancer (Figure 4-4).

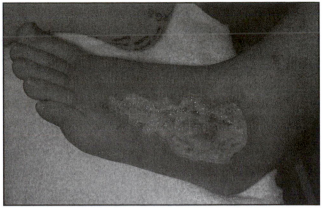

Figure 4-4. Full-thickness infected wound on the dorsal aspect of the left foot. (See this figure in the Color Atlas following page 39.)

PHYSICAL THERAPIST EXAMINATION

HISTORY

♦ General demographics: Mr. Dawson is a 37-year-old male whose primary language is English. He is right-hand dominant and has a high school diploma and completed trade school.

♦ Social history: He lives with his second wife. He has two children who live with his first wife but stay with him every other weekend.

♦ Employment/work: Mr. Dawson is an electrician. He has not worked in the past 3 months due to illness.

♦ Living environment: He lives in a one-story house that has been made wheelchair accessible.

♦ General health status
  • General health perception: Mr. Dawson reports that his health status is poor.
  • Physical function: He reports that his physical function is extremely limited.
  • Psychological function: He reports being depressed over his health status, inability to work, lack of mobility, and word finding problems. He reports frequent nightmares and sleep disturbances.
  • Role function: Husband, father, financial provider.
  • Social function: His social activities have been limited for the past 2 months due to illness.

♦ Social/health habits: Mr. Dawson is a social drinker, and he smokes marijuana occasionally. He and his wife are independent with the HEP that the physical therapist gave to them in the rehabilitation unit. The HEP is designed to improve his balance, coordination, and ambulatory endurance.

♦ Family history: Unknown.

♦ Medical/surgical history: He was diagnosed with brain cancer 5 months ago. He has had surgical resection of the tumors 3 months ago and is completing his final round of chemotherapy. Mr. Dawson has had two seizures since surgery but none in the past month.

♦ Current condition(s)/chief complaint(s): His wife reports that his main problems are a nonhealing foot wound and inability to communicate effectively. His wife also reports that he developed cellulitis in the LLE about 3 months ago during his hospital stay. The wound developed a few weeks later. She feels the wound was made worse by his earlier problems with incontinence and lack of mobility. He was discharged from the inpatient rehabilitation unit yesterday due to a plateau in functional improvements. While on the unit he received the following interventions: speech therapy to assist with communication, occupational therapy to assist with dressing and feeding and to enable compensation for the loss of use of his left upper extremity (LUE) due to upper motor neuron damage, and physical therapy for mobility and exercises to improve his strength and coordination. Wound care at this time consisted of saline irrigation, silver sulfadiazine, two gauze pads, and gauze wrap changed three to four times per day pending wound drainage. Outpatient speech therapy will be started after the initial physical therapy examination.

♦ Functional status and activity level: Mr. Dawson is now independently mobile with a quad cane both indoors and for short community outings, including shopping or going to football games. He has no functional use of his LUE.

♦ Medications: Methylprednisolone, carmustine, hydrocodone, furosemide, cephalexin, transdermal fentanyl, lorazepam, phenytoin.

♦ Other clinical tests
  • Wound cultures during his acute care admission revealed an *Enterobacter* infection.

- However, recent wound culture was positive for *Staphylococcus aureus* infection only.
- The following laboratory test results are available from the patient's medical record (see Table 3-10)
  - Hgb=10.5 g/dL
  - Hct=30%
  - Total lymphocyte count=1400/mm^3
  - Fasting blood glucose=130 mg/dL
  - Serum albumin=3.7 g/dL
  - Serum prealbumin=18.0 mg/dL
  - Serum transferrin=180 mg/dL
  - Urine glucose=Negative
  - Blood urea nitrogen (BUN)=12.0 mg/dL
  - Creatinine=0.9 mg/dL

SYSTEMS REVIEW

- ◆ Cardiovascular/pulmonary
  - BP: 149/87 mmHg
  - Edema: Present left greater than right ankle
  - HR: 88 bpm
  - RR: 15 bpm
- ◆ Integumentary
  - Presence of scar formation: None
  - Skin color: Periwound erythema
  - Skin integrity: Open wound dorsal lateral left foot
- ◆ Musculoskeletal
  - Gross range of motion: BLE WNL for patient's age
  - Gross strength: Impaired distal LLE, absent LUE
  - Gross symmetry: Asymmetrical
  - Height: 6'2" (1.88 m)
  - Weight: 171 lbs (77.57 kg)
- ◆ Neuromuscular
  - Transfers/transitions: Independent, requires RUE assist
  - Gait: Independent with quad cane on the right
  - Gross coordination: Impaired LLE, absent LUE
- ◆ Communication, affect, cognition, language, and learning style
  - Communication, affect, cognition
    - He is oriented to name, place, and situation but not to time
    - He frequently has word finding problems and answers questions inappropriately
    - He defers questions regarding health, treatments, and home environment to his wife
    - He cried on three occasions during the physical therapy examination
  - Learning barriers: Mr. Dawson has impaired cognition and communication, and Mrs. Dawson has none
  - Learning preferences: He learns best by demonstra-

tion and repetition, while his wife has no learning preferences

TESTS AND MEASURES

- ◆ Anthropometric characteristics
  - BMI=22
  - Normal BMI ranges from 18.5 to 24.9[37]
- ◆ Assistive and adaptive devices: Quad cane and manual wheelchair
- ◆ Circulation
  - Pulse exam[38-40] (see Table 3-4)
    - Performed as an indicator of arterial blood flow
    - Popliteal, DP and PT arteries=2+ B
  - Capillary refill[41-47] (see Table 3-5)
    - Performed as an indicator of superficial blood flow
    - Capillary refill time was 2 seconds bilaterally
  - ABI[45,47-57] (see Table 3-6)
    - Performed to identify the presence of arterial insufficiency and assist with determining if compression therapy would be contraindicated
    - ABI=0.9 bilaterally
  - Homans' sign[81-84] (see Table 3-8)
    - Performed as a screening procedure on patients with suspected peripheral vascular disease to identify the presence of a DVT because of the potentially devastating consequences of a DVT (eg, pulmonary embolism)
    - Homans' was negative bilaterally
    - Alternative: Because of the potentially devastating consequences of a DVT (eg, pulmonary embolism) and the poor reliability of the Homans' sign, the reader is referred to the scoring system developed by Anand for an alternate screening strategy that more accurately predicts the presence of a DVT[84,85]
  - Venous filling time[47] (see Table 3-13)
    - Performed to identify the presence of venous insufficiency and assist with determining the plan of care
    - R=12 seconds and L=11 seconds
- ◆ Cranial and peripheral nerve integrity
  - Semmes-Weinstein monofilament testing
    - Performed to identify his ability to detect the potentially harmful effects of trauma or pressure
    - He is unable to detect 5.07 monofilament on the majority of the LLE
- ◆ Integumentary integrity
  - Associated skin
    - Skin color: Periwound erythema extending 1.2 cm from wound edge
    - Hair growth: Normal

- Nail growth: Normal
- Temperature: Periwound and left foot are warmer than right to palpation
- Texture/turgor: Normal
- Edema: Figure-of-eight R=53.2 cm and L=56.0 cm[107]
  - Activities, positioning, and postures that produce or relieve trauma to the skin
    - Mr. Dawson prefers to lay on his left side
  - Wound
    - Irregular-shaped, open wound noted left dorsal, lateral foot
    - Full-thickness wound measures 14.2 cm x 8.1 cm, depth 0.4 cm
    - Wound bed: 95% covered with adherent yellow slough
    - Wound drainage: Copious, thick, purulent
- Muscle performance
  - Left ankle=4/5
  - Left knee=4+/5
  - LUE absent
- Pain
  - Because Mr. Dawson was unable to use a 0 to 10 numeric pain scale, he was presented with a series of facial expressions to describe his foot pain
  - He points to the face with a neutral expression for pain[92-94]
- Range of motion
  - Ankle dorsiflexion: R=0 to 15 degrees, L=0 to 13 degrees
- Self-care and home management
  - Self-care
    - During the interview Mrs. Dawson reports that her husband requires assistance with bathing and dressing
    - He also requires cues for safety (eg, to turn off the stove after heating up food)
- Sensory integrity
  - Proprioception
    - Decreased in left foot, ankle, and knee
    - Absent LUE
- Work, community, and leisure integration or reintegration
  - Work
    - He is unable to work due to his current medical condition
    - Mr. Dawson believes that he is able to drive
  - Leisure
    - He continues to enjoy watching television and movies

EVALUATION

Mr. Dawson's history and risk factors previously outlined indicate that he has decreased mobility, left leg motor function, sensation, absent LUE function, and impaired cognition and communication due to brain cancer. He is immunocompromised, on the borderline of malnutrition, and at risk for impaired wound healing.[108-111] He has a nonhealing, infected full-thickness wound and impaired immune response. He has limitations in self-care.

DIAGNOSIS

Although Mr. Dawson continues to have impairments in his LUE and LLE motor function, is no longer able to ambulate without an assistive device, and has limitations in self-care, the improvements in these impairments and functional limitations have plateaued with previous rehabilitation. While small gains may continue to be made over time with continuation of his HEP, physical therapy interventions at this time will be directed toward his integumentary impairment. Mr. Dawson has a nonhealing, infected full-thickness skin involvement wound and scar formation. He has impaired: circulation; cranial and peripheral nerve integrity; integumentary integrity; muscle performance; range of motion; and sensory integrity. He is functionally limited in self-care and home management and in work, community, and leisure actions, tasks, and activities. These findings are consistent with placement in Pattern D: Impaired Integumentary Integrity Associated With Full-Thickness Skin Involvement and Scar Formation. These impairments and functional limitations will be addressed in determining the prognosis and the plan of care.

PROGNOSIS AND PLAN OF CARE

Over the course of the visits, the following mutually established outcomes have been determined:
- Edema is reduced
- Knowledge of behaviors that foster healthy habits, wellness, and prevention is increased
- Patient/family knowledge and awareness of diagnosis, prognosis, interventions, and anticipated goals and outcomes are increased
- Risk factors are reduced
- Risk of secondary impairment is reduced
- Skin integrity is restored
- Tissue perfusion and oxygenation are enhanced
- Tolerance to positions and activities is increased

To achieve these outcomes, the appropriate interventions for this patient are determined. These will include: coordination, communication, and documentation; patient/client-related instruction; therapeutic exercise; functional training in self-care and home management; functional training in work, community, and leisure integration or reintegration; integumentary repair and protection techniques; electrotherapeutic modalities; and physical agents and mechanical modalities.

Based on the diagnosis and prognosis, Mr. Dawson is expected to require between 12 to 28 visits over a 4-week period of time. Mr. Dawson lives with his wife, is depressed, is immunocompromised, and his mobility and self-care have plateaued with inpatient rehabilitation. He is impaired and is in relatively poor health.

INTERVENTIONS

RATIONALE FOR SELECTED INTERVENTIONS

Therapeutic Exercise

Exercise is important for this patient since impairments exist in his ankle AROM. He is also to continue the HEP that he received from the rehab unit, since Mr. Dawson may continue to make slow improvements in his mobility and strength. Ankle AROM exercises performed in combination with leg elevation may assist with edema control.[112]

Integumentary Repair and Protection Techniques

Integumentary repair and protection techniques will be important for this patient. Sharp debridement will be performed since it decreases the risk of infection, reduces bacterial concentration within the wound bed, and improves the bactericidal activity of leukocytes. It also shortens the inflammatory phase of wound healing, decreases the energy required for wound healing, and eliminates a physical barrier to wound healing by removing dead tissue and debris.[100-102]

After communication with his referring physician, topical lidocaine gel will be used to decrease the pain of debridement.[112] Gentamicin sulfate 0.1% will also be effective against *Staphylococci,* and the wound culture report revealed that his specific infection was susceptible to this antimicrobial.

An alginate was chosen to absorb wound drainage and prevent periwound maceration.[71,72,113,114] A gauze dressing was chosen due to the presence of infection and need for frequent dressing changes.[71,72]

Given his ABI of 0.9, a short-stretch compression bandage will also be used to assist with edema control without compromising tissue perfusion.

Electrotherapeutic Modalities

Since Mr. Dawson is immunocompromised and has a nonhealing, infected wound that has failed to heal with conservative wound management, adjunctive interventions, such as electrical stimulation, are warranted to enhance wound healing. Electrical stimulation may assist with wound heal-

ing by: restoring normal skin current; producing galvanotaxis; stimulating proliferation and function of macrophages, fibroblasts, platelets, endothelial cells, and keratinocytes; increasing blood flow; increasing bactericidal function of neutrophils and macrophages; reducing edema; and facilitating debridement. High voltage current was chosen because the majority of research on the use of electrical stimulation to enhance wound healing has employed this technique. Negative polarity was chosen to assist with decreasing wound infection.[115-130]

Physical Agents and Mechanical Modalities

Pulsatile lavage with suction has been selected for this patient because of its beneficial effects. It removes loosely adhered debris, bacteria, exudate, and residual topical agents. It softens eschar, facilitates debridement, and hydrates the wound bed, promoting moist wound healing. The negative pressure of pulsatile lavage may enhance granulation tissue formation, epithelialization, and local tissue perfusion. It may also decrease pain associated with wound management techniques. Pulsatile lavage with suction is preferable to whirlpool because it does not require dependent positioning.[74,105,106,115,131-134]

COORDINATION, COMMUNICATION, AND DOCUMENTATION

Communication will occur with Mrs. Dawson to assist with her husband's care at home and to encourage support for him. Communication will occur with his primary care physician and oncologist to assist with the management of infection, to monitor his overt medical condition, and to assist with pain control as needed. A referral to a registered dietitian will be recommended to monitor his nutritional status and maximize wound healing. Communication will occur with the speech therapist to assist with patient communication and to reinforce speech therapy goals. If Mr. Dawson consents or if his affect does not improve, a psychological consult may be warranted. All elements of the patient's management will be documented.

PATIENT/CLIENT-RELATED INSTRUCTION

Mr. and Mrs. Dawson will be instructed in wound management and methods to limit factors that adversely affect wound healing. Particular emphasis will be placed on:
- Understanding that open wounds or inappropriately bandaged wounds provide a direct pathway for bacteria to enter the body, increasing the risk of infection and sepsis
- Knowing that dressings with strike-through or that are seeping must be changed
- Instructing the patient and his wife in the signs and symptoms of worsening infection and action plan if these occur

♦ Instructing the patient and his wife in proper wound management
♦ Avoiding skin trauma by:
  ● Being aware of potential obstacles, such as furniture that, if bumped against, may further traumatize wound
  ● Protecting against excessive heat or cold (bath water, heating pads, and environmental)
  ● Not using any topical agents on the skin or wound unless directed to do so by a clinician
  ● Instructing Mrs. Dawson in twice daily skin inspection of the LUE and LLE to assess for signs of trauma, irritation, or excessive pressure
♦ Providing her with written copies of instructional material, HEP, and self-care techniques, since a significant amount of information is being presented to Mrs. Dawson, and she verbalizes a considerable amount of emotional stress in coping with his illness

THERAPEUTIC EXERCISE

♦ Strength, power, and endurance training
  ● Active ankle pumps
    ■ 20 repetitions
    ■ Three or more times per day
    ■ Preferably performed with LEs elevated above the level of the heart

FUNCTIONAL TRAINING IN SELF-CARE AND HOME MANAGEMENT

♦ Self-care
  ● Mrs. Dawson will be instructed in ways to help her husband position his leg during sleep and rest to avoid pressure on the dorsal, lateral aspect of his left foot
    ■ Discourage sleeping on his left side
    ■ Prop LEs when sitting to decrease edema
    ■ Pillows can be used to prevent left hip external rotation while lying supine or when propping the extremity to avoid pressure on the lateral aspect of his left foot
  ● To prevent worsening of his wound infection, his wife will be instructed to cover his bandage in a plastic bag when bathing to prevent further wound contamination
  ● Mrs. Dawson will be shown how to perform skin checks to identify early signs of the adverse effects of pressure or trauma on areas with decreased sensation
  ● He will be encouraged to take frequent short walks to enhance circulation and decrease peripheral edema

FUNCTIONAL TRAINING IN WORK, COMMUNITY, AND LEISURE INTEGRATION OR REINTEGRATION

♦ Leisure
  ● Proper positioning to decrease edema and pressure on Mr. Dawson's lateral left foot while watching television will be encouraged

INTEGUMENTARY REPAIR AND PROTECTION TECHNIQUES

♦ Debridement: Selective
  ● The yellow adherent slough will be selectively debrided with a scalpel, forceps, and scissors as able
  ● If pain is produced with debridement, a physician's order will be requested for a 2% lidocaine gel that can be applied to the wound prior to debridement
♦ Dressings
  ● A calcium alginate will be applied to his wound
  ● A gauze pad will be placed over the alginate and secured with a 6-ply roll gauze
  ● A short stretch compression bandage will be applied from the MTPs to the proximal tibial
♦ Topical agents
  ● Gentamicin sulfate 0.1% will be applied to the wound bed

ELECTROTHERAPEUTIC MODALITIES

♦ Electrical stimulation
  ● After pulsatile lavage with suction and any additional debridement has been completed, a saline-moistened gauze will be placed within the wound bed, covered with a carbon electrode, and secured in place with tape or a Velcro wrap
  ● A similarly prepared electrode will be secured to his distal lower leg 15 to 20 cm proximal to the wound
  ● Electrical stimulation parameters
    ■ Frequency: 80 to 125 Hz
    ■ Interpulse interval: 50 to 100 microseconds
    ■ Polarity: Negative
    ■ Stimulation intensity: 75 to 200 volts
      ▸ Intensity may produce a comfortable paresthesia, however, given his sensory deficits, this may not be reliable indicator of intensity
      ▸ In which case, a submotor intensity that is less than or equal to 200 volts should be used
    ■ Duration: 45 minutes
    ■ Frequency: 3 to 7 days per week

PHYSICAL AGENTS AND MECHANICAL MODALITIES

♦ Hydrotherapy: Pulsatile lavage
  • Mr. Dawson will be positioned comfortably supine with his left leg elevated slightly on pillows
  • After removing the dressings, his LE will be placed on moisture-impermeable padding to absorb any irrigant runoff
  • The irrigant, 1000 mL of normal saline, should be warmed to approximately 98° to 100°F to maintain wound normothermia[70,135]
  • The physical therapist will wear appropriate personal protective equipment including, but not necessarily limited to, clean gloves, a face shield, hair covering, foot coverings, and a moisture-impermeable gown
  • The wound will be thoroughly irrigated using pulsatile lavage with an irrigation pressure of 4 to 8 psi
  • After treatment, the intact skin will be dried with a towel and any necessary sharp debridement should be performed prior to electrical stimulation

ANTICIPATED GOALS AND EXPECTED OUTCOMES

♦ Impact on pathology/pathophysiology
  • Debridement of all nonviable tissue is achieved within 2 weeks.
  • Edema is resolved with positioning and dressings within 2 weeks.
  • Periwound erythema is resolved within 2 weeks.
  • Tissue perfusion and oxygenation are enhanced.
  • Wound size is reduced to <8.0 x 6.0 cm without purulent drainage in 4 weeks.
♦ Impact on impairments
  • Circulation is enhanced.
  • ROM is increased in the left ankle.
  • Sensory awareness is increased.
  • Wound drainage is controlled with dressings and positioning to require only daily dressing changes in two visits.
♦ Impact on functional limitations
  • Tolerance to positions or activities is increased.
♦ Risk reduction/prevention
  • Risk factors are reduced.
  • Risk of secondary impairment is reduced.
  • Self-management of symptoms is improved.
♦ Impact on health, wellness, and fitness
  • Disability is reduced.
  • Health status is improved.
♦ Impact on societal resources
  • A referral is made for a psychologist or psychiatrist if the patient's emotional status has not improved in 2 weeks.
  • A referral is made for a registered dietician within 1 week.
  • Resources are utilized in a cost-effective way.
  • Utilization of physical therapy services is optimized.
♦ Patient/client satisfaction
  • Care is coordinated with patient, wife, speech therapist, oncologist, and other health care professionals.
  • Documentation occurs throughout patient management and follows APTA's *Guidelines for Physical Therapy Documentation*.[80]
  • Patient and caregiver knowledge and awareness of the diagnosis, prognosis, interventions, and anticipated goals and outcomes are increased.
  • Patient and caregiver understanding of anticipated goals and expected outcomes is increased.

REEXAMINATION

Reexamination is performed throughout the episode of care.

DISCHARGE

Mr. Dawson is discharged from physical therapy after a total of 20 physical therapy sessions and attainment of his goals and expectations. These sessions have covered his entire episode of care. He is discharged because he has achieved his goals and expected outcomes.

PSYCHOLOGICAL ASPECTS

Mr. Dawson has a significant life-altering illness, brain cancer. He continues to have functional limitations of his LUE and LLE and continues to have significant impairments in communication. To maximize compliance and outcomes, his wife and family will be involved in all aspects of his care. The assistance of a psychologist or psychiatrist may be beneficial. It is imperative that all members of the health care team work synergistically to maximize outcomes and patient/family satisfaction, particularly with this medically complex patient.

REFERENCES

1. American Diabetes Association. Consensus development conference on diabetic foot care. *Diabetes Care.* 1999;22(8):1354-1360.
2. Porth CM. *Pathophysiology: Concepts of Altered Health States.* 5th ed. Philadelphia, Pa: Lippincott-Raven Publishers; 1998.
3. Nolte MS, Karam JH. Pancreatic hormones and antidiabetic drugs. In: Katzung BG, ed. *Basic and Clinical Pharmacology.*

New York, NY: Lange Medical Books/McGraw-Hill; 2001:711-734.

4. Miller JW, Kraemer FB. Endocrine and metabolic disorders: diabetes mellitus. In: Carruthers SG, Hoffman BB, Melmon KL, Nierenberg DW, eds. *Melmon and Morrelli's Clinical Pharmacology.* 4th ed. New York, NY: McGraw-Hill; 2000:529-644.

5. Meyer JS. Diabetes and wound healing. *Crit Care Nurs Clin North Am.* 1996;8(2):195-201.

6. Campbell RK, White JR. Insulin therapy in type 2 diabetes. *J Am Pharm Assoc.* 2002;42(4):602-611.

7. Bild DE, Selby JV, Sinnock P, Browner P, Showstack JA. Lower extremity amputation in people with diabetes. *Diabetes Care.* 1989;12(1):24-31.

8. Drazin B, Melmed S, LeRoith D, eds. Complications of diabetes. *Molecular and Cellular Microbiology of Diabetes Mellitus.* Vol III. New York, NY: Alan R Liss, Inc; 1989.

9. Sakamoto N, Alberti KG, Hotta N, eds. *Pathogenesis and Treatment of NIDDM and Its Related Problems.* Amsterdam, The Netherlands: Excepta Medica; 1994.

10. Cohen MP. *The Polyol Paradigm and Complications of Diabetes.* New York, NY: Springer-Verlag; 1987.

11. Bensen WE, Brown GC. *Diabetes and Its Ocular Complications.* Philadelphia, Pa: WB Saunders Co; 1988.

12. American Diabetes Association. Preventive foot care in people with diabetes. *Diabetes Care.* 2002;25(Suppl 1):S69-S70.

13. Sims DS, Cavanagh PR, Ulcrecht JS. Risk factors in the diabetic foot: recognition and management. *Phys Ther.* 1988;68(12):1887-1901.

14. Most RS, Sinnock P. The epidemiology of lower extremity amputations in diabetic individuals. *Diabetes Care.* 1983;6(1):87-91.

15. Ramsey SD, Newton K, Blough D, et al. Incidence, outcomes, and cost of foot ulcers in patient with diabetes. *Diabetes Care.* 1999;22:382-387.

16. Snyder RJ. Offloading difficult wounds and conditions in the diabetic foot. *Ostomy/Wound Management.* 2002;48(1):22-35.

17. Birke JA, Patout CA Jr, Foto JG. Factors associated with ulceration and amputation in the neuropathic foot. *J Orthop Sports Phys Ther.* 2000;30:91-97.

18. Mueller MJ. Identifying patients with diabetes mellitus who are at risk for lower extremity complications: use of Semmes-Weinstein monofilaments. *Phys Ther.* 1996;76(1):68-71.

19. Mueller MJ. Etiology, evaluation and treatment of the neuropathic foot. *Crit Rev Phys Rehabil Med.* 1992;3(4):289-309.

20. Laing P. Diabetic foot ulcers. *Am J Surg.* 1994;167(Suppl 1A):31S-36S.

21. Pham H, Armstrong DG, Harvey C, Harkless LB, Giurini JM, Veres A. Screening techniques to identify people at high risk for diabetic foot ulceration: a prospective multi-center trial. *Diabetes Care.* 2000;23:606-611.

22. Duckworth T, Boulton A, Betts R, Franks C, Ward J. Plantar pressure measurements and the prevention of ulceration in the diabetic foot. *J Bone Joint Surg.* 1985;67B(1):79-85.

23. Banks AS, McGlamry ED. Charcot foot. *J Am Podiatr Med Assoc.* 1989;79(5):213-235.

24. Edmonds ME. The neuropathic foot in diabetes: part I: blood flow. *Diabetes Med.* 1986;3:111-115.

25. Rosenberg CS. Wound healing in patients with diabetes mellitus. *Nurs Clin North Am.* 1990;25(1):247-261.

26. American Diabetes Association. Diabetic retinopathy. *Diabetes Care.* 2002;25(Suppl 1):S90-S93.

27. Myers BA. *Wound Management: Principles and Practice.* Upper Saddle River, NJ: Prentice Hall; 2004.

28. American Diabetes Association. Implications of the United Kingdom Prospective Diabetes Study. *Diabetes Care.* 2002;25(Suppl 1):S28-S32.

29. American Diabetes Association. Implications of the Diabetes Control and Complications Trial. *Diabetes Care.* 2002;25(Suppl 1):S25-S27.

30. Snyder RJ, Cohen MM, Sun C, Livingston J. Osteomyelitis in the diabetic patient: overview, diagnosis, microbiology. *Ostomy/Wound Management.* 2001;47(1):18-30.

31. Jelinek J, Levy E. Radiologic considerations for the diabetic extremity. In: Kominski SJ, ed. *Medical and Surgical Management of the Diabetic Foot.* St. Louis, Mo: Mosby-Yearbook; 1994:145-160.

32. Sage R. Surgery in the infected foot. In: Kominski SJ, ed. *Medical and Surgical Management of the Diabetic Foot.* St. Louis, Mo: Mosby-Yearbook; 1994:279-300.

33. Thompson PD, Smith DJ Jr. What is infection? *Am J Surg.* 1994;167(1A):7S-11S.

34. Levine JM, Totolos E. A quality-oriented approach to pressure ulcer management in a nursing facility. *Gerontologist.* 1994;34(3):413-417.

35. Stotts NA, Wipke-Tevis D. Co-factors in impaired healing. *Ostomy/Wound Management.* 1996;42(2):44-53.

36. Hutchinson JJ, Lawrence LC. Wound infection under occlusive dressings. *J Hosp Infect.* 1991;17:83-94.

37. Franklin BA, ed. *American College of Sports Medicine's Guidelines for Exercise Testing and Prescription.* 6th ed. Philadelphia, Pa: Lippincott Williams & Wilkins; 2000.

38. Lewis CD. Peripheral arterial disease of the lower extremity. *J Cardiovasc Nurs.* 2001;15(4):45-63.

39. Blank CA, Irwin GH. Peripheral vascular disorders: assessment and intervention. *Nurs Clin North Am.* 1990;25(4):777-794.

40. Ward K, Schwartz ML, Thiele R, Yoon P. Lower extremity manifestations of vascular disease. *Clin Podiatr Med.* 1998;15(4):629-672.

41. Schriger D, Baraff L. Defining normal capillary refill: variation with age, sex, and temperature. *Ann Emerg Med.* 1988;17(9):932-935.

42. Strozik K, Pieper C, Cools F. Capillary refill time in newborns: optimal pressing time, site of testing and normal values. *Acta Paediatr.* 1998;87(3):310-312.

43. Bates-Jensen BM. Chronic wound assessment. *Nurs Clin North Am.* 1999;34(4):799-845.

44. Gorelick MH, Shaw KN, Murphy KO. Validity and reliability of clinical signs in the diagnosis of dehydration in children. *Pediatrics.* 1997;99(5):e6.

45. Collins KA, Sumpio BE. Vascular assessment. *Clin Podiatr Med Surg.* 2000;17(2):171-191.

46. McGee SR, Boyko EJ. Physical examination and chronic lower-extremity ischemia: a critical review. *Arch Intern Med.* 1998;158:1357-1364.

47. Doughty DB, Waldrop J, Ramundo J. Lower-extremity ulcers of vascular etiology. In: Bryant RA, ed. *Acute and Chronic Wounds: Nursing Management.* St. Louis, Mo: Mosby; 2000.

48. Cameron J. Arterial leg ulcers. *Nurs Standard.* 1996;10(26):50-56.

49. Carpenter JP. Noninvasive assessment of peripheral vascular occlusive disease. *Advances in Skin and Wound Care.* 2000;13(2):84-85.

50. Rubano JJ, Kerstein MD. Arterial insufficiency and vasculitides. *J Wound Ostomy Continence Nurs.* 1998;25(3):147-157.

51. Fiegelson H, Criqui MH, Fronek A, Langer R, Molgaard C. Screening for peripheral arterial disease: the sensitivity, specificity, and predictive value of noninvasive tests in a defined population. *Am J Epidemiol.* 1994;140(6):426-534.

52. Leng G, Fowkes F, Lee A, Dunbar J, Housley E, Ruckey C. Use of ankle brachial pressure index to predict cardiovascular evens and death: a cohort study. *BMJ.* 1996;313:1440-1443.

53. Cantwell-Gab K. Identifying chronic peripheral arterial disease. *Am J Nurs.* 1996;96(7):40-47.

54. Sloan H, Wills EM. Ankle-brachial index: calculating your patient's vascular risk. *Nursing.* 1999;29(10):58-59.

55. Jaffe MR. Diagnosis of peripheral arterial disease: utility of the vascular laboratory. *Clin Cornerstone.* 2002;4(5).

56. Dillavou E, Kahn MB. Peripheral vascular disease: diagnosing and treating the 3 most common peripheral vasculopathies. *Geriatrics.* 2003;58(2):37-42.

57. American Diabetes Association. Peripheral arterial disease in people with diabetes. *Diabetes Care.* 2003;26(12):3333-3341.

58. Bell-Krotoski J, Tomancik E. The repeatability of testing with Semmes-Weinstein monofilaments. *J Hand Surg.* 1987;12A(1):155-161.

59. Edelman D, Sanders LJ, Pogach L. Reproducibility and accuracy among primary care providers of a screening examination for foot ulcer risk among diabetic patients. *Prev Med.* 1998;27(2):274-278.

60. Caselli A, Phaum H, Giurini JM, Armstrong DG, Veres A. The forefoot-to-rearfoot plantar pressure ratio is increased in severe diabetic neuropathy and can predict ulceration. *Diabetes Care.* 2002;25:1066-1071.

61. Birke JE, Cornwall MW, Jackson M. Relationship between hallux limitus and ulceration of the great toe. *J Orthop Sports Phys Ther.* 1988;10(5):172-176.

62. Fernando DJ, Masson EA, Veves A, Boulton AJ. Relationship of limited joint mobility to abnormal foot pressures and diabetic foot ulcerations. *Diabetes Care.* 1991;14(1):8-11.

63. Bandy W, Irion J. The effect of time on static stretching on the flexibility of hamstring muscles. *Phys Ther.* 1994;74(9):845-852.

64. Dunbar CC, Robertson RJ, Baun R, et al. The validity of regulating exercise intensity by ratings of perceived exertion. *Med Sci Sports Exerc.* 1992;24(1):94-99.

65. Brown HE, Mueller MJ. A "Step-to" gait decreases pressures on the forefoot. *J Orthop Sports Phys Ther.* 1998;28(3):139-145.

66. Kwon OY, Mueller MJ. Walking patterns used to reduce forefoot plantar pressures in people with diabetic neuropathies. *Phys Ther.* 2001;81(2):828-835.

67. Green MF, Aliabadi Z, Green BT. Diabetic foot: evaluation and management. *South Med J.* 2002;95(1):95-101.

68. Bolton LL, Monte K, Pirone LA. Moisture and healing: beyond the jargon. *Ostomy/Wound Management.* 2000;46(1A):51S-62S.

69. Eaglstein WH, Falanga V. Chronic wounds. *Surg Clin North Am.* 1997;77(3):689-700.

70. Evans RB. An update on wound management. *Frontiers Hand Rehabil.* 1991;7(3):409-432.

71. McCulloch JM. Decision point: wound dressings. *PT Magazine.* 1996;4(5):52-62.

72. Maklebust J. Using wound care products to promote a healing environment. *Crit Care Nurs Clin North Am.* 1996;8(2):141-158.

73. Bergstrom N, Bennett MA, Carlson CE, et al. *Treatment of Pressure Ulcers: Clinical Practice Guideline No. 15.* Rockville, Md: US Department of Health and Human Services. Agency for Health Care Policy and Research; December 1994. AHCPR Publication No. 95-0652.

74. Barr JE. Principles of wound cleansing. *Ostomy/Wound Management.* 1995;41(7A):15S-22S.

75. Kato H, Takada T, Kawamura T, Hotta N, Toril S. The reduction and redistribution of planter pressures using foot orthoses in diabetic patients. *Diabetes Res Clin Pract.* 1996;31(1-3):115-118.

76. Albert A, Rinoie C. Effect of custom orthotics on plantar pressure distribution in the pronated diabetic foot. *J Foot Ankle Surg.* 1994;33(6):598-604.

77. American Diabetes Association. Implications of the diabetes control and complications trial. *Diabetes Care.* 1999;22(Suppl 1):S24-S25.

78. American Diabetes Association. Smoking and diabetes. *Diabetes Care.* 2002;25(Suppl 1):S80-S81.

79. Brannon FJ, Foley MW, Starr JA, Black MG. *Cardiopulmonary Rehabilitation: Basic Theory and Application.* 2nd ed. Philadelphia, Pa: FA Davis Co; 1993.

80. American Physical Therapy Association. Guide to physical therapist practice. 2nd ed. *Phys Ther.* 2001;81:9-744.

81. Goodman CC, Boissonault WG. *Pathology: Implications for the Physical Therapist.* Philadelphia, Pa: WB Saunders Co; 1998.

82. Magee DJ. *Orthopedic Physical Assessment.* 3rd ed. Philadelphia, Pa: WB Saunders Co; 1997:638.

83. Urbano F. Homans' sign in the diagnosis of deep vein thrombosis. *Hosp Phys.* 2001;March:22-24.

84. Anand SS, Wells PS, Hunt D, Brill-Edwards P, Cook D, Ginsberg JS. Does this patient have a deep vein thrombosis? *JAMA.* 1998;279(14):1094-1099.

85. Ofri D. Diagnosis and treatment of deep vein thrombosis. *West J Med.* 2000;173:194-197.

86. VanSwearingen JM, Brach JS. Making geriatric assessment work: selecting useful measures. *Phys Ther.* 2001;81:1233-1252.

87. VanSwearingen JM, Paschal KA, Bonino P, Yang J. The modified gait abnormality rating scale for recognizing the risk of recurrent falls in community-dwelling adults. *Phys Ther.* 1996;76:994-1002.

88. Wolfson L, Whipple R, Anmerman P, Tobin JN. Gait assessment in the elderly: a gait abnormality rating scale and its relation to falls. *Journal of Gerontology.* 1990;45(1):M12-M19.

89. Steffen TM, Hacker TA, Mollinger L. Age-and gender-related test performance in community-dwelling elderly people: six-minute walk test, Berg balance scale, timed up and go test, and gait speeds. *Phys Ther.* 2002;82:128-137.

90. Thornbahn L, Newton R. Use of the Berg balance test to predict falls in elderly persons. *Phys Ther.* 1996;76(6):576-585.

91. Harada N, Chiu V, Damron-Rodriguez J, Fowler E, Siu A, Reuben DB. Screening for balance and mobility impairment in elderly individuals living in residential care facilities. *Phys Ther.* 1995;75:462-469.

92. Ferraz M, Quaresma M, Aquino L, Atra E, Tugwell P, Goldsmith C. Reliability of pain scales in the assessment of literate and illiterate patients with rheumatoid arthritis. *J Rheumatol.* 1990;17(8):1022-1024.

93. Hoher J, Munster A, Klein J, Eypasch E, Tilling T. Validation and application of a subjective knee questionnaire. *Knee Surg Sports Traumatol Arthrosc.* 1995;3(1):26-33.

94. Paice JA, Cohen FL. Validity of a verbally administered numeric rating scale to measure cancer pain intensity. *Cancer Nurs.* 1997;20(2):88-93.

95. Wolf SL, Barnhart HX, Kutner NG, McNeely E, Coogler C, Xu T. Reducing frailty and falls in older persons: an investigation of Tai Chi and computerized balance training. *J Am Geriatr Soc.* 1996;44:489-497.

96. Wolf SL, Barnhart HX, Ellison GL, Coogler C. The effect of Tai Chi Quan and computerized balance training on postural stability in older subjects. *Phys Ther.* 1997;77:371-382.

97. Mulrow CD, Gerety MB, Kanten D. A randomized trial of physical rehabilitation for very frail nursing home residents. *JAMA.* 1994;271:519-524.

98. Harada N, Chiu V, Fowler B, Lee M, Reuben DB. Physical therapy to improve functioning of older people in residential care facilities. *Phys Ther.* 1995;75:830-839.

99. Tinetti ME, Baker DI, McAvay G. A multifactorial intervention to reduce the risk of falling among elderly people living in the community. *N Engl J Med.* 1994;331:821-827.

100. Singhal K, Reis G, Kerstein MD. Options for nonsurgical debridement of necrotic wounds. *Advances in Skin and Wound Care.* 2001;14(2):96-103.

101. Sieggreen MY, Maklebust J. Debridement: choices and challenges. *Advances in Skin and Wound Care.* 1997;10(2):32-37.

102. Troyer-Caudle J. Debridement: removal of non-viable tissue. *Ostomy/Wound Management.* 1993;39(6):24-32.

103. Ovington LG. Wound care products: how to choose. *Advances in Skin and Wound Care.* 2001;14(5):224-232.

104. Sprung P, Hou Z, Ladin DA. Hydrogels and hydrocolloids: an objective product comparison. *Ostomy/Wound Management.* 1998;44(1):36-53.

105. McCulloch J, Boyd VB. The effects of whirlpool and dependent position on lower extremity volume. *J Orthop Sports Phys Ther.* 1992;16(4):169-173.

106. McCulloch JM. Physical modalities in wound management: ultrasound, vasopneumatic devices, hydrotherapy. *Ostomy/Wound Management.* 1995;41(5):30-37.

107. Pugia ML, Middel CJ, Seward SW, et al. Comparison of acute swelling and function in subjects with lateral ankle injury. *J Orthop Sports Phys Ther.* 2001;31:384-388.

108. Guenter P, Malyszek R, Zimmaro D, et al. Survey of nutritional status in newly hospitalized patients with stage III or stage IV pressure ulcers. *Advances in Skin and Wound Care.* 2000;13(4):164-168.

109. Bobel LM. Nutritional implications in the patient with pressure sores. *Nurs Clin North Am.* 1987;22(2):379-390.

110. Skipper A. *Dietician's Handbook of Enteral and Parenteral Nutrition.* 2nd ed. Gaithersburg, Md: Aspen Publications; 1998.

111. Telfer NR, Moy RL. Drug and nutrient aspects of wound healing. *Dermatol Clin.* 1993;11(4):729-735.

112. Smith S, Hall C, Brody LT. The ankle and foot. In: Hall CM, Brody LT, eds. *Therapeutic Exercise: Moving Toward Function.* Philadelphia, Pa: Lippincott Williams & Wilkins; 1999:489.

113. Margolis S, ed. *The John's Hopkins Consumer Guide to Drugs.* New York, NY: Medletter Associates, Inc; 2002.

114. Fanucci D, Seese J. Multi-facetted use of calcium alginates. *Ostomy/Wound Management.* 1991;37:16-22.

115. Thomas S. Use of calcium alginate dressings. *Pharm J.* 1985;235:188-190.

116. Houghton PE, Kincaid CB, Lovel M, et al. Effect of electrical stimulation on chronic leg ulcer size and appearance. *Phys Ther.* 2003;83(1):17-28.

117. Houghton PE, Campbell KE. Choosing an adjunctive therapy for the treatment of chronic wounds. *Ostomy/Wound Management.* 1999;45(8):43-52.

118. Devine P. Electrical stimulation and wound healing. *J Wound Ostomy Continence Nurs.* 1998;25(6):291-295.

119. Houghton PE, Kincaid CB, Lovell M, et al. PL-RR-220-F: effect of electrical stimulation on chronic leg ulcers. *Phys Ther.* 2000;80(5):S71.

120. Broussard CL, Mendez-Eastman S, Frantz RA. Adjuvant wound therapies. In: Bryant RA, ed. *Acute and Chronic Wounds: Nursing Management.* 2nd ed. St. Louis, Mo: Mosby; 2000.

121. Kincaid CB, Lavoie KH. Inhibition of bacterial growth in vitro following stimulation with high voltage, monophasic, pulsed current. *Phys Ther.* 1989;69(8):651-655.

122. Kloth LC, McCulloch JM. Promotion of wound healing with electrical stimulation. *Advances in Skin and Wound Care.* 1996;9(5):42-45.

123. Cukjati D, Robnik-Sikonja M, Rebersek S, Kononenko I, Miklavcic D. Prognostic factors, prediction of chronic wound healing by electrical stimulation. *Med Biol Eng Comput.* 2001;39(5):542-550.

124. Mawson AR, Siddiqui FH, Connolly BJ, et al. Effect of high voltage pulsed galvanic stimulation on sacral transcutaneous oxygen levels in the spinal cord injured. *Paraplegia.* 1993;31(5):311-319.

125. Franek A, Polak A, Kucharzewski M. Modern application of high voltage stimulation for enhanced wound healing of venous ulceration. *Med Eng Phys.* 2000;22(9):647-655.

126. Griffin JW, Tooms RE, Mendius RA, Clifft JK, Vander Zwag RV, El-Zeky F. Efficacy of high volt pulsed current for healing pressure ulcers in patients with spinal cord injury. *Phys Ther.* 1991;71(6):433-444.

127. Gilcreast DM, Stotts NA, Froelicher ES, Baker LL, Moss KM. Effect of electrical stimulation on foot skin perfusion in persons with or at risk for diabetic foot ulcers. *Wound Repair Regen.* 1998;6(5):434-441.

128. Fitzgerald GK, Newsome D. Treatment of a large infected thoracic spine wound using high voltage pulsed monophasic current. *Phys Ther.* 1993;73(6):355-360.

129. Szuminsky NJ, Albers A, Unger P, Eddy J. Effect of narrow, pulsed high voltages on bacterial viability. *Phys Ther.* 1994;74(7):660-667.

130. Jacques PF, Brogan MS, Kalinowski DP. High-voltage electrical treatment of refractory dermal ulcers. *Physician Assistant.* 1997;21(3):84-97.

131. Mulder GD. Treatment of open-skin wounds with electrical stimulation. *Arch Phys Med Rehabil.* 1991;72(6):375-377.

132. Morgan D, Hoelscher J. Pulsed lavage: promoting comfort and healing in home care. *Ostomy/Wound Management.* 2000;46(4):44-49.

133. Luedtke-Hoffman K, Shafer DS. Pulsed lavage in wound cleansing. *Phys Ther.* 2000;80(3):292-300.

134. Loehne HB. Pulsatile lavage with concurrent suction. In: Sussman C, Bates-Jensen BM, eds. *Wound Care: A Collaborative Practice Manual for Physical Therapists and Nurses.* 2nd ed. Gaithersburg, Md: Aspen Publications; 2001:643-660.

135. Scott RG, Loehne HB. Treatment options: 5 questions: and answers: about pulsed lavage. *Advances in Skin and Wound Care.* 2000;13(3):133-134.

Impaired Integumentary Integrity Associated With Skin Involvement Extending Into Fascia, Muscle, or Bone and Scar Formation (Pattern E)

Katherine Biggs Harris, PT, MS
Jenna Driscoll, PT, MS

INTRODUCTION

Impaired integumentary integrity that is associated with skin involvement into fascia, muscle, or bone with scar formation is a challenge for physical therapists. These wounds extend beyond the fascia and will heal by repair since there will not be any dermal appendages remaining in the wound bed to assist with repopulation of epithelial tissue. Repair of deep wounds that extend beyond the fascia may occur in a variety of ways. Small wounds may be allowed to granulate, contract, and re-epithelialize from the periphery, or larger defects may be surgically repaired with the use of skin grafts or flaps.

Many diseases and injuries can cause a wound that extends beyond the fascia. These include: burn injuries (thermal or electrical), traumatic injuries, tumors, neuropathic ulcers, pressure ulcers, and vascular ulcers to name a few. Vascular ulcers and neuropathic ulcers have been discussed in Pattern C: Impaired Integumentary Integrity Associated With Partial-Thickness Skin Involvement and Scar Formation and Pattern D: Impaired Integumentary Integrity Associated With Full-Thickness Skin Involvement and Scar Formation. This chapter will focus on burns, traumatic injuries, and pressure ulcers.

Because these deeper wounds will heal with scar, the physical therapist will also need to address potential impair-ments of the musculoskeletal and neuromuscular systems. Depending on the extent of deficits, a patient may fall into more than one diagnostic pattern. According to the *Guide* the assigning of a diagnostic label will assist the therapist in determining the prognosis and the plan of care. For patients with injuries that extend to muscle, tendon, and bone there may be additional diagnostic labels that should be used in conjunction with the integumentary pattern.[1] For example, if a patient sustained an open fracture he or she may best be placed in both Pattern E: Impaired Integumentary Integrity Associated With Skin Involvement Extending Into Fascia, Muscle, or Bone and Scar Formation and Musculoskeletal Pattern G: Impaired Joint Mobility, Muscle Performance, and Range of Motion Associated With Fracture. Depending on the severity or complexity of the examination and evalua-tion, the patient may be classified into either one or both of the above patterns.

ANATOMY

The anatomy of muscle, tendon, and bone has been thoroughly discussed within the musculoskeletal practice patterns. When these structures are exposed the physi-cal therapist must recognize whether they appear normal or necrotic. Healthy muscles in general appear a deep red color due to the significant vascular supply. Muscles that

	Table 5-1	
WOUND CLOSURE TERMINOLOGY COMPARISON		
Type of Closure	*Description*	*Examples*
Primary Intention (Also called primary healing and first intention)	A. Closure by direct approximation, use of sutures or steri-strips, pedicle flap, or skin graft B. Direct approximation	Surgical incisions and lacerations
Delayed Primary Healing or Closure	A. Closure after several days but prior to granulation tissue evident in the wound	
Secondary Intention (Also called spontaneous healing, second intention, or tertiary closure)	A. Wound is left open to heal spontaneously either by epithelialization or granulation, contraction, and epithelialization B. Surgical closure after granulation tissue is present in the wound bed or spontaneous healing	Contaminated wounds Partial-thickness wounds
Tertiary Intention (Also called tertiary healing or third intention)	A. Delayed healing after several days, occurs after granulation tissue is noted in the wound bed B. A combination between primary and secondary intention, also called delayed primary closure	Amputation site, dehisced wound

have begun to necrose may appear gray or brown. Tendons normally exhibit a glossy sheen. When tendons begin to disintegrate they become grayish and separate into thin fibrous strands. Bones normally have a shiny smooth appearance, but when damaged can appear gray to black in color and have irregular surfaces.[2]

PHYSIOLOGY

Wounds heal through a three-phase overlapping process that allows for wound closure.[2-5] Wound closure may also be described as "healing by intention."[6] Healing by intention has been described as primary healing or first intention, spontaneous healing or secondary intention, and tertiary healing or third intention. The last has also been referred to as delayed primary closure. There have been some changes to this terminology. Currently healing has been described as primary healing or closure, delayed primary healing or closure, or secondary healing or closure. Secondary closure has been broken into two categories: spontaneous healing and surgical closure after granulation tissue is present in the wound.[2,5,6] Table 5-1 offers a comparison of wound closure and healing terminology.

Wound closure, whether from delayed primary healing, secondary healing by surgical repair, or tertiary healing,

offers the potential for physical therapists to work with patients who have had skin grafts and/or flaps for soft tissue wound coverage. Goals of soft tissue coverage include: wound closure, revascularization to injured soft tissue and bone, and prevention of infection and potential bony nonunion as a result of bone ischemia.[6] Split-thickness skin grafts (STSGs) are composed of epidermis and a varying portion of dermis and are used to cover deep partial- or full-thickness wounds.[6,7] STSGs vary in depth from very thin to thick depending on the dermatome (a microsurgical instrument utilized to procure skin grafts of various depths) used and can be from 10 to 25 thousandths of an inch thick.[7]

A skin graft is skin that is separated completely from its "bed," and the resultant wound is referred to as the donor site. The skin graft is then transplanted to the recipient site or wound area. Skin grafts may be autografts, allografts, or xenografts. Autografts are skin grafts that are transferred from one part of a patient's body to another part of his or her own body. Allografts are donated cadaver skin and are also known as homografts. Xenografts are skin obtained from a different species, such as porcine skin.[6,7] For the purposes of this chapter skin grafts will refer to autografts. Additional information regarding allografts and xenografts may be found in the surgical literature.

STSGs may be utilized on large surface areas of skin loss

and granulating tissue beds, and they may be either sheet grafts or meshed grafts. Sheet grafts offer a more cosmetic appearance after maturation and have less scar formation than meshed grafts. Meshed grafts are used to cover greater surface areas when available skin for grafting is less than the area in need of coverage. Meshed grafts also offer contourability to joint areas and may allow for drainage immediately postoperatively.[5-7]

Full-thickness skin grafts (FTSGs) include the epidermis and all of the dermis. These are utilized for small areas of full-thickness loss, such as fingertip or eyelid injuries or burns, where durability and cosmesis are of utmost importance.[6,7]

Initial graft survival depends on diffusion of nutrition, also known as plasma imbibition, from the recipient site. Revascularization, through either spontaneous reconnection of blood vessels of the recipient site and the skin graft or via growth of new vessels (neovascularization) from the recipient site into the graft, generally occurs within 3 to 5 days, the proliferative phase of healing. Skin graft viability is dependent on revascularization from the recipient site and low bacterial level.[6] Bacteria levels that exceed 10^5 organisms/gram of tissue have been implicated in skin graft failure and delayed wound healing.[5,6] Skin graft loss is commonly the result of hematoma or seroma under the graft, friction or shear forces applied to the graft (such as that which may occur with patient mobilization), poor vascularity, or infection.[6]

Skin flap coverage transfers tissue from one area to another with an intact vascular supply. Flaps utilized for wound coverage may consist of skin, subcutaneous tissue, fascia, and/or muscle.[6-8] Flaps may also include tendon, bone, or other tissue, such as the omentum,[6] but these flaps will not be covered in this text. This text will cover flaps classified as random pattern, axial pattern, or musculocutaneous flaps.

Random flaps that sustain their blood supply using the dermal and subdermal plexus are further categorized as rotation flaps or advancement flaps. Most rotation flaps are created when tissue is incised on three sides, undermined, and rotated into the wound defect. The donor area is then closed, primarily with sutures or skin grafts. A different type of random rotation flap is the transposition flap. In this flap, tissue is moved either over or under intervening normal tissue. Examples include the Z-plasty or W-plasty often used in plastic surgery to correct scar contracture. Advancement flaps are created when tissue is raised, undermined, and then pushed or pulled into the wound defect. Again the donor site is closed with sutures or a skin graft. The two primary techniques utilized in this procedure are V-Y advancement or bipedicle advancement.[6,8,9] Additional information regarding these techniques can be located in the plastic surgery literature.

Axial pattern flaps carry both an artery and a vein when relocated. Vascularity is derived from specific arterial flow that is identifiable in the subcutaneous tissue. These flaps may be transferred over a great anatomical distance and may be used as a "free flap." A free flap is removed from one location along with its artery and vein and placed into the defect. Once in its new location the vessels are re-anastomosed using microvascular surgical techniques. Forms of axial flaps include the peninsular flap, where skin, subcutaneous tissue, and vessels are removed, or the island flap, where only the subcutaneous tissue and vessels are removed. Should an island free flap be used, coverage with a STSG will be necessary. Once more the donor area will be closed via suturing or skin grafting.[6,8,9]

Musculocutaneous flaps are comprised of skin, subcutaneous tissue, and muscle. These flaps receive blood supply from the muscle that provides a rich vascular supply to areas with impaired vascularity. As a side note, once the muscle is removed from its original site, it no longer functions.[6-8] Physical therapist considerations regarding potential impairments associated with muscle flap procedures must be addressed during the examination and evaluation. Musculocutaneous flaps offer several distinct advantages over skin flaps, including enhanced vascular supply, provision of padding (especially over bony prominences), and presence of sensation in the flap skin. These flaps may also be used as rotated flaps or free flaps.[6-9]

PATHOPHYSIOLOGY

Pressure ulcers, especially ulcers that extend beyond the fascial plane, account for a significant number of wounds that require surgical closure.[2,6,9] Pressure ulcers are staged based on tissue destruction depth.[2-4,10] The staging system, originally put forth by the NPUAP, was based on the early work of Shea.[2] Stage I pressure ulcers are defined as areas of nonblanchable erythema of intact skin. In individuals with dark toned skin the areas may be represented by a purplish-blue discoloration, local warmth, edema, or induration. Stage II pressure ulcers are defined as superficial ulcers that have a shallow crater or blister. Stage III ulcers, defined as deep craters, may have evidence of undermining, but the destruction depth may extend to, but not through, the fascia. Finally, Stage IV pressure ulcers are deep ulcers with extensive necrosis that may extend to muscle, tendon, and bone. As pointed out by Myers,[2] the staging system put forth by the NPUAP does not consistently fall into the categories as defined in the *Guide*.[1] This is also seen when using burn injury depth or Wagner's neuropathic wound classification. Unfortunately, there is no universal classification system that transcends all wounds and can be used by all disciplines. It is imperative that physical therapists fully understand the nomenclature in any given environment.

For the most part, pressure ulcer formation is preventable. Risk factors associated with pressure ulcer formation include: age, friction and shear forces, moisture (incontinence, sweat),

	Table 5-2		
Burn Depth of Injury and Presentation Classifications			
Superficial	*Partial-Thickness Superficial*	*Partial-Thickness Deep*	*Full-Thickness*
First Degree	*Second-Degree Superficial*	*Second-Degree Deep*	*Third-Degree*
Superficial, involves the epidermis	Superficial partial-thickness, involves the epidermis and the papillary dermis	Deep partial-thickness, involves the epidermis and reticular dermis	Full-thickness, involves the epidermis, dermis, subcutaneous tissue, and potentially beyond
No integumentary disruption	Blisters usually present	Blisters usually disrupted	No blisters
Red in appearance	Moist appearance Erythema Edema Pain	Red and white in appearance Positive capillary refill Decreased sensation Pain	White, brown, or black in appearance Absent capillary refill Asensate
May involve tissue desquamation	Heals via regeneration	May heal via regeneration if dermal appendages remain in adequate numbers or heal via repair, scar formation is possible	Healing occurs via repair, usually surgical Scarring

activity, mobility, nutrition, and sensation.[2,4,11,12] These risk factors appear in a number of risk assessment tools, including the Braden Scale for Pressure Sore Risk[13] that was discussed in Pattern A: Primary Prevention/Risk Reduction for Integumentary Disorders. A number of hypothesized risk factors exist that are not always assessed including: low diastolic pressure, use of multiple medications, educational level, low socioeconomic status, and the availability of support systems.[2]

Burn injuries (thermal, chemical, or electrical) may also result in full-thickness injuries that extend to muscle, tendon, and bone. When examining thermal injuries, one needs to address the amount and extent of tissue destruction that is often based on the temperature of the offending agent and the time exposed to the offending agent.[14] Burn size is described as the total body surface area (TBSA) of involved skin. A rough TBSA estimate for adults is calculated using the Rule of 9's[15,16] and for children using the Lund and Browder chart.[17] Originally, burns were classified as first degree, second degree, or third degree based on depth of tissue destruction. First-degree injuries, such as sunburn, involve the epidermis. Second-degree burns are subclassified as either superficial or deep partial-thickness depending on the depth of dermal injury. A burn with an intact blister

would be considered a superficial second-degree injury, while a burn with a ruptured blister could be considered a deep second-degree injury. Third-degree burns are full-thickness and, depending on the time and temperature of the offending agent, can extend beyond the fascial plane. People caught in house or car fires for a long period of time would most likely display third-degree burns. For the most part, this classification system has been replaced by the terms superficial, partial-thickness, and full-thickness.[14] Table 5-2 provides information regarding depth of injury associated with burns and the two classification systems.

Electrical injuries may be low voltage electrical injuries that usually occur in the home or high voltage injuries that usually occur in the workplace.[18] Electrical injuries often result in deeper tissue destruction due to the fact that electricity follows the path of least resistance. Tissue resistance increases from nerve to vessel, to muscle, to skin, to tendon, to fat, and finally to bone, resulting in internal tissue damage.[19] Electrical injuries typically have both an entrance wound, the part of the body the electricity enters the body, and an exit wound, the point the electricity exits the body to find its ground.[18] The cutaneous injury can appear somewhat inconsequential but soft tissue and muscle damage can result in significant tissue defects requiring surgical repair.[18,19] The physical therapist treating patients with electrical injuries should also look for possible cardiopulmonary impairments, renal involvement, spinal cord damage, and vascular damage. These additional deficits will become evident during the examination process and could potentially necessitate the use of two practice patterns.

Wounds that extend into deeper tissues are a potential breeding ground for either endogenous or exogenous bacteria. Endogenous bacteria include *Staphylococcus aureus* and *Pseudomonas aeruginosa* (both normally found on the skin) and *Escherichia coli* (normally found in the intestinal tract). Exogenous microbes include *Pseudomonas aeruginosa* and *aspergillus* both normally found in the environment. Clinical signs of wound infection include pain, erythema, edema, warmth, and drainage.[2-5] Physical therapists must consider wound drainage during their examination. Wound cultures can be obtained in order to identify the amount and type of bacteria present (see Pattern D: Impaired Integumentary Integrity Associated With Full-Thickness Skin Involvement and Scar Formation for information regarding tissue biopsy and fluid aspiration).

IMAGING/CLINICAL TESTS

Imaging and clinical tests are detailed in Pattern D: Impaired Integumentary Integrity Associated With Full-Thickness Skin Involvement and Scar Formation.

PHARMACOLOGY

The following pharmacological agents may be utilized, in the management of patients with deep integumentary injuries, to enhance healing.

- ◆ Antibiotics
  - Examples: Penicillins, cephalosporins, vancomycin, gentamicin
  - Actions: Inhibit bacterial growth
  - Administered: Oral or parenteral
  - Side effects:
    - Hypersensitivity reactions, GI upset, secondary infections, ototoxicity, and nephrotoxicity
    - Ototoxicity and nephrotoxicity are rare
- ◆ Pain medications
  - Examples: NSAIDs, Demerol, Percocet, codeine, morphine
  - Actions: Anti-inflammatory effects, analgesic effects, platelet effects
  - Administered: Oral or parenteral
  - Side effects: Gastric intolerance, tinnitus, tolerance and dependence
- ◆ Topical antimicrobials (ointments)
  - Examples: Gentamicin, bacitracin, Betadine

- Actions: Inhibit bacterial growth
- Side effects:
  - Hypersensitivity reactions, secondary infections, nephrotoxicity, and ototoxicity
  - As above nephrotoxicity and ototoxicity are rare unless utilized in large volumes
- ◆ Topical antimicrobials (creams)
  - Examples: Silver sulfadiazine, mafenide acetate, nitrofurazone, nystatin
  - Actions: Inhibit bacterial and fungal growth
  - Side effects: Hypersensitivity reactions, leukopenia, secondary infections
- ◆ Topical antimicrobials (solutions)
  - Examples: Silver nitrate, acetic acid, sodium hypochlorite, mafenide acetate, bacitracin (many of these preparations will need to be made in the institution's pharmacy based on patient need and physician preference)
  - Actions: Inhibit bacterial growth
  - Side effects: Hypersensitivity reactions, acidosis

Case Study #1:
Post-Traumatic Soft Tissue Wound Extending to Bone With *Aspergillus* Infection

Tom White is a 27-year-old male who has a large, traumatic open wound on the right thigh extending into bone (Figures 5-1 through 5-3).

PHYSICAL THERAPIST EXAMINATION

HISTORY

- ◆ General demographics: Tom White is a 27-year-old black American male whose primary language is English. He is right-hand dominant.
- ◆ Social history: He is married and has two young children (ages 3 and 8 years).
- ◆ Employment/work: The patient is a forklift operator. His wife reports that he has recently been taking computer and accounting classes at a local community college in order to change occupation in the near future.
- ◆ Living environment: Mr. White and his family live in a one-level, second-floor apartment with one flight of stairs without a railing. Eviction is pending.
- ◆ General health status
  - General health perception: His wife reports that he

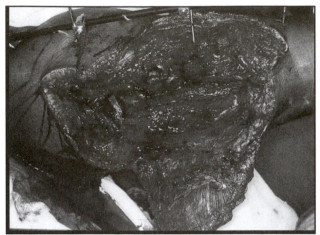

Figure 5-1. Right lateral thigh wound operative debridement and external fixator placement. (See this figure in the Color Atlas following page 39.)

is in excellent health. He has no remarkable medical or surgical history.

- Physical function: Normal for his age of 27 years.
- Psychological function: Normal per his wife. Therapist unable to screen initially due to sedation.
- Role function: Forklift operator, student, husband, father.
- Social function: He enjoys basketball and staying fit.

♦ Social/health habits: Mr. White does not smoke or abuse IV drugs. His wife does report occasional use of marijuana and alcohol.

♦ Family history: Unknown.

♦ Medical/surgical history: No prior hospitalizations.

♦ Current condition(s)/chief complaint(s): Two weeks prior to physical therapist examination, Tom White was involved in a high-speed motorcycle crash during which he was thrown off of his motorcycle into a wooded area. He was admitted to our acute care hospital via the emergency room as a "full trauma." He was immediately intubated, sedated, and resuscitated in the surgical intensive care unit. Positive loss of consciousness was reported.

♦ Hospital course: Patient underwent the following surgeries prior to physical therapist examination (chronological order):

- E-lap, ligation of profunda artery and vein, abdominal wall debridement, bilateral femoral external fixation, radical debridement right thigh wound, bilateral chest tube and naso-gastric tube placement
- Repeat debridement of abdominal wall and skin/muscle/bone right thigh, revision of right femur external fixator, intramedullary (IM) rodding left femur fracture

- Third debridement of right thigh wound and placement of antibiotic beads
- Fourth debridement of right thigh wound and split-thickness skin graft to edges of wound (in effort to decrease wound size)
- External fixator removal and IM rodding right femur
- Removal of IM rod right femur (due to signs of infection) and replacement of external fixator
- Latissimus dorsi flap to right femur wound
- Debridement of failed free flap right femur wound (day before physical therapy exam)

♦ Functional status and activity level: Prior to injury, Mr. White was independent with all functional activities. His wife reports that he has been physically active and enjoys basketball, football, and working out at a local gym. She admits that he also enjoys racing his motorcycle.

♦ Medications: Patient was not taking any medications prior to admission.

- At time of physical therapist examination the following medications are being administered: Subcutaneous (SQ) heparin, gentamicin, Pepcid, morphine, propofol, Ativan

♦ Other clinical tests

- Initial Glasgow Coma scale=15
- Initial diagnostic imaging studies as follows:
  - Head CT: Negative
  - Spine films: Negative
  - Transesophageal echocardiogram (TEE): Negative for aortic arch injury
  - Pelvic/LE angiogram: Bleeding of right profunda artery and vein
  - Extremity films/exam:
    - Open Grade III B[20] right femur fracture with large soft tissue deficit, visible bone comminution, and gross contamination
    - Mangled Extremity Severity Score (MESS)=6 (Table 5-3)
      - Is a scale that was developed to assist with decisions of limb salvage vs amputation
      - The MESS is based on skeletal/soft tissue injury, ischemia time, hypotension, and age
      - Literature has indicated that a score of 7 points or less is nearly always compatible with a salvageable limb[21]
    - Closed left femur fracture
  - Abdominal CT scan
    - Grade III liver laceration
    - Left colonic mesentery tear
    - Multiple small bowel contusions

Table 5-3

MANGLED EXTREMITY SEVERITY SCORE

MESS Classification	Points
Skeletal/Soft Tissue Injury	
Low velocity (stab, simple fracture)	1
Medium energy (open/multiple fractures, dislocation)	2
High energy (close-range shot gun or high velocity GSW, crush)	3
Very high energy (above + gross contamination, soft tissue avulsion)	4
Limb Ischemia (score doubled for ischemia >6 hours)	
Pulse reduced or absent, perfusion normal	1
Pulseless, paresthesias, diminished capillary refill	2
Cool, paralyzed, insensate	3
Shock	
Systolic BP >90 mmHg	0
Hypotension transiently	1
Persistent hypotension	2
Age	
<30 years	0
30 to 50 years	1
>50 years	2

- Lab values
  - Hct=29% indicating anemia
  - WBC=15,000/mm^3 indicating infection
  - ESR=25 mm/hr indicating inflammation and possibly a marker for infection
  - Platelets=250,000/mm^3 (WNL)

SYSTEMS REVIEW

- Cardiovascular/pulmonary
  - BP: 110/60 mmHg
  - Edema: 3+ pitting edema RLE, 2+ pitting edema LLE
  - HR: 110 bpm
  - RR: 22 bpm (mechanically ventilated on synchronized intermittent mandatory ventilation [SIMV] mode)
- Integumentary
  - Presence of scar formation: None
  - Skin color: Can be difficult to assess in black American patients, however skin of the proximal RLE observed to be darker than all other extremities
  - Skin integrity
    - Open abdominal wound (extending to fascia—fascia closed)
    - Large open wound on lateral right thigh (extending to bone)
- Musculoskeletal
  - Gross range of motion
    - RLE deficits at hip, knee, and ankle
    - LLE deficits in knee flexion
  - Gross strength: Difficult to assess because of level of sedation, however suspicious for deficit right anterior tibialis due to position of foot and lack of spontaneous ankle dorsiflexion
  - Gross symmetry: Not assessed
  - Height: 6'0" (1.83 m)
  - Weight: 185 lbs (83.92 kg)
- Neuromuscular
  - Difficult to assess due to level of sedation/bedrest
- Communication, affect, cognition, language, and learning style
  - Limited communication due to sedative medication
  - Intermittent command following and verbal expression of pain
  - Appropriately nodding "yes/no" during more alert moments
  - Per interview with patient's wife, he is able to read and write English

TESTS AND MEASURES

- ♦ Circulation
  - Capillary refill: Right foot 3 seconds, left foot 2 seconds
  - Pulses: Right DP pulse diminished, left normal
- ♦ Cranial and peripheral nerve integrity
  - Difficult to assess due to level of sedation
- ♦ Integumentary integrity
  - Associated skin
    - Skin of right foot dehydrated and cracked and heel red, positive blanching
    - Posture of RLE in hip external rotation, placing pressure on skin of right lateral leg and foot
    - Edema=3+ pitting right foot, 2+ pitting left foot
    - RLE warm to palpation
  - Wound
    - Location: Right lateral thigh
    - Size: 35x30 cm, depth centrally to bone 20 cm
    - Tunnels/tracts: Proximally toward hip 8 cm, distally toward knee 5 cm
    - Photography: Grid not accurate due to large size, photo taken to document wound appearance
    - Tissue: 50% red granulation, 40% viable red/pink muscle, 10% gray-green cottony residue over slough surrounding exposed femur
    - Anatomical structures: Exposed femur bone at fracture site, vastus lateralis with large tissue deficit, rectus femoris, biceps femoris
    - Drainage: Minimal serous drainage with green-blue tinge
    - Odor: Foul odor present
    - Related information: Low grade fever with spikes to 101° to 102°F
    - Signs of infection: Above noted
      - ▸ Physical therapist recommends to physician that tissue cultures be performed to diagnose wound infection and to guide physical therapy and medical intervention
      - ▸ Once the signs of infection are recognized and a patient has not responded to a standard wound management regime, steps should be taken to identify the infecting organism and determine whether it is bacterial or fungal[22]
      - ▸ Once identified, the appropriate treatment approach may be employed
      - ▸ Two methods for culturing open wounds most commonly used by physical therapists: Swab cultures and quantitative tissue cultures
        - ○ Swab cultures are considered to be of questionable value because multiple bacteria are present in wound fluid and on the wound surface
        - ○ Surface organisms do not correlate well with the number and type of organisms present in wound tissue
        - ○ Quantitative tissue cultures give a more accurate indication of the infecting organism(s) because an actual piece of wound tissue is cultured and analyzed by a microbiologist
        - ○ This test determines the type of organism and the number of colonies per gram of tissue
        - ○ A wound is considered "infected" if that number is $\geq 10^5$ microorganisms[3]
        - ○ The quantitative tissue culture/biopsy of the right lateral thigh wound tissue revealed $>10^5$ *Enterobacter* and *Aspergillus* fumigatus

- ♦ Muscle performance: Functional muscle testing was performed as patient was unable to undergo manual muscle testing due to decreased level of alertness
  - UEs: Spontaneous movement noted in all muscle groups
  - LEs
    - RLE revealed no active hip or quadriceps contraction, trace hamstring contraction, no active dorsiflexion
    - LLE revealed active movement in all muscle groups, possible weakness in quadriceps group
- ♦ Pain
  - Unable to verbalize pain level for use of numeric pain rating scale
  - Positive facial grimace and gestures, as well as slightly increased HR with RLE movement suggestive of pain response
- ♦ Range of motion: Measured with goniometer
  - Hip flexion: R=40 degrees and L=80 degrees
  - Hip abduction: R=15 degrees and L WNL
  - Hip internal rotation: R=-10 degrees and L=0 degrees
  - Knee flexion: R=10 degrees and L=60 degrees
  - Ankle dorsiflexion: R=-10 degrees and L WNL
- ♦ Sensory integrity
  - Positive limb movements to deep palpation and to noxious stimulation
- ♦ Ventilation and respiration/gas exchange
  - RR: Increased during exam from 22 to 28 bpm
  - Ventilator support: Presently on SIMV mode, noted to be taking some spontaneous breaths supported by ventilator
  - Airway clearance: Unable to independently clear secretions requiring frequent suctioning through endotracheal (ET) tube

EVALUATION

Tom White is a 27-year-old previously healthy male who has been examined 2 weeks after a motorcycle crash. Mr. White sustained multiple traumatic injuries and has resultant impairments in all four systems reviewed. The RLE demonstrates significant integumentary impairment. He is at risk for permanent loss of RLE function as there are also impairments in sensation, ROM, and strength. Mr. White is currently unable to perform any functional activities or ADL due to his physical and medical conditions.

Due to the size and severity of open wound, Mr. White is at high risk for secondary impairments including repeated wound infection. Because of the medical diagnosis of *Aspergillus* infection based on culture results, he is also at risk for further soft tissue destruction. *Aspergillus* is the most common fungal cause of invasive soft tissue infection.[23] Like other fungi, it is found in the environment in moist, warm, dirty areas and was probably contracted by Mr. White via his open femur fracture when he landed in the woods.[24] When examining Mr. White's wound, fungal elements (green-gray, cottony) could be seen in the debris and nonviable tissue, indicating new fungal growth. Once the body has been invaded by *Aspergillus*, the infection can spread across tissue planes and hematogenously. This is the reason that early diagnosis and debridement of involved tissue are so important.[25,26] The high contamination level of Mr. White's initial wound and the delay in diagnosis of Aspergillosis until time of physical therapy examination may adversely affect the viability of his right leg.

DIAGNOSIS

Mr. White has a large infected wound with skin involvement extending to the bone and has pain. He has impaired: circulation; cranial and peripheral nerve integrity; integumentary integrity; muscle performance; range of motion; sensory integrity; and ventilation and respiration/gas exchange. He is functionally limited in actions, tasks, and activities. Although the impairments stated are described under three different Preferred Practice Patterns (Musculoskeletal Pattern I: Impaired Joint Mobility, Motor Function, Muscle Performance, and Range of Motion Associated With Bony or Soft Tissue Surgical Procedures; Cardiovascular/Pulmonary Pattern F: Impaired Ventilation/Respiration With Mechanical Ventilation Secondary to Respiratory Failure; and Pattern E: Impaired Integumentary Integrity Secondary to Skin Involvement Extending Into Fascia, Muscle, or Bone and Scar Formation), the necessary interventions and anticipated goals and outcomes make these findings consistent with placement at this time in Pattern E: Impaired Integumentary Integrity Associated With Skin Involvement Extending Into Fascia, Muscle,

or Bone and Scar Formation.[1] These impairments and functional limitations will be addressed in determining the prognosis and the plan of care.

PROGNOSIS AND PLAN OF CARE

Over the course of the visits, the following mutually established outcomes have been determined:
♦ Debridement of nonviable tissue is achieved and wound size is reduced and eventually closed
♦ Muscle performance is increased
♦ Patient is able to ambulate with appropriate assistive device and within weightbearing precautions specified by orthopaedic surgeon
♦ Patient is able to perform activities related to self-care and home management
♦ Pain is decreased
♦ Physical function is improved
♦ Placement needs are determined
♦ Wound is free from infection and prepared for surgical closure

To achieve these outcomes, the appropriate interventions for this patient are determined. These will include: coordination, communication, and documentation; patient/client-related instruction; therapeutic exercise; functional training in self-care and home management; prescription, application, and, as appropriate, fabrication of devices and equipment; integumentary repair and protection techniques; and physical agents and mechanical modalities.

Based on the diagnosis and prognosis, Mr. White is expected to require between 60 to 80 visits over a 16-week period of time. Mr. White is severely impaired with comorbidities, complications, and secondary impairments.

INTERVENTIONS

RATIONALE FOR SELECTED INTERVENTIONS

Therapeutic Exercise

Patients with traumatic integumentary injury involving structures at or below the dermal level are at risk for scar tissue formation. This process involves soft tissue contraction that can result in joint contracture. Tom White also had the pathology of bony fracture status post surgical stabilization. These combined factors place him at high risk for soft tissue shortening and joint contracture, indicating to the physical therapist the need for a comprehensive therapeutic exercise program. Although there is a lack of literature addressing exercise in patients with wounds, articles in the area of burn care suggest that a combination of passive, active, and active-assistive exercise in appropriate directions inhibit contracture formation.[27]

Prescription, Application, and, as Appropriate, Fabrication of Devices and Equipment

As described above, Mr. White is at risk for contracture development. The use of positioning devices can assist in maintaining optimal soft tissue length and joint integrity, facilitating maximal return to function. Mr. White's edema will also be managed with appropriate positioning and the use of compression bandages in order to facilitate RLE function.[27] Edema reduction has been noted to enhance wound and soft tissue healing.[2]

Integumentary Repair and Protection Techniques

Due to the presence of infection, wound cleansing techniques are indicated. Hydrotherapy was available and is known as one of the most commonly applied modalities for wound cleansing.[3] Since the wound culture results indicated *Aspergillus* infection, the decision was made not to use hydrotherapy in order to prevent facilitation of fungal growth. Fungi like wet, moist places. Alternative wound cleansing and debridement techniques were utilized and will be described.

The selection of which dressings and topical solution to utilize for cleansing is based on the clinical findings of wound examination, the culture results, and communication with the infectious disease specialists. For treatment of Aspergillosis, the infectious disease specialists have recommended intravenous (IV) amphotericin B for 6 weeks.

Physical Agents and Mechanical Modalities

A literature review has revealed the usefulness of amphotericin B lavage or direct installation in some patients although this method has not been prospectively studied as extensively as the IV form of therapy has been.[26] In the literature, there is documentation of the efficacy of bladder irrigation with amphotericin B for *Aspergillus* urinary tract infection (UTI) and of transthoracic intracavitary instillation of amphotericin B for pulmonary Aspergillosis. This was well tolerated by all patients without toxicity.[28] It has therefore been decided that directly treating the femur bone (including medullary canal) and wound tissue with amphotericin B may be an effective adjunct to IV therapy.

COORDINATION, COMMUNICATION, AND DOCUMENTATION

Communication directly with Mr. White will initially be limited due to his impaired level of alertness. Communication initially regarding his physical impairments and functional limitations will be directed toward his

family and nursing staff. Communication and coordination of his care with nursing, medical staff, and occupational therapy will also be essential. Due to the complexity of his case, continuous discussion with various consulting physicians (orthopaedic surgeons, general surgeons, plastic surgeons, and infectious disease specialists) will need to occur. All communication will be documented in the medical record. The therapist will collaborate with the case manager on discharge planning.

PATIENT/CLIENT-RELATED INSTRUCTION

Education will be initially directed toward the patient's family and nursing staff due to the patient's inability to participate in learning. His wife and primary nurse will be educated regarding the current state of his impairments and functional limitations and in specific techniques to increase LE ROM and decrease edema. The physical therapist will also educate these individuals on elements of infection control procedures related to RLE open wound.

THERAPEUTIC EXERCISE

- Balance, coordination, and agility training: Initiated as appropriate
- Flexibility exercises
  - Stretching exercises should be done after warming up, using a slow and steady stretch accompanied by deep breathing, and building hold up to 30 seconds
  - RLE hip flexion, hip abduction, hip internal rotation, knee flexion, and ankle dorsiflexion
  - LLE knee flexion
  - Patient's wife will play a key role in assisting patient with stretching exercises several times per day
- Gait and locomotion training: Initiated as appropriate
- Strength, power, and endurance training
  - Patient will be instructed in ventilatory muscle exercise with focus on decreased support required from ventilator and increased cough strength
  - Begin at the lowest level possible by asking patient to actively contract LE musculature during AAROM as able
  - LE strengthening may be modified in future after further tests and measures are performed

FUNCTIONAL TRAINING IN SELF-CARE AND HOME MANAGEMENT

- Self-care
  - ADL training in bed will be initiated as soon as appropriate
    - Bathing/grooming
    - Use of trapeze
    - Bed mobility/rolling/scooting

- ■ Transfer training
- Safety awareness training with LE weightbearing limitation of "Touch-Down" with external fixator in place (per orthopaedic surgeon)

PRESCRIPTION, APPLICATION, AND, AS APPROPRIATE, FABRICATION OF DEVICES AND EQUIPMENT

- ♦ Adaptive devices
  - Mr. White will be provided with a hospital bed, low air loss mattress, and trapeze system
- ♦ Assistive devices
  - He will be provided with a walker for use during transfer training
  - Parallel bars may be used for standing and gait training
- ♦ Orthotic devices
  - The physical therapist will fabricate a custom posterior right ankle and foot splint
  - The ankle joint will be positioned as near to neutral as possible and the heel will be off-loaded
  - A bar will be attached to the splint laterally to encourage positioning out of external rotation
- ♦ Supportive devices
  - Short stretch compression bandages will be applied to both LEs in order to manage edema
  - Pillows will be utilized under RLE to also manage edema

INTEGUMENTARY REPAIR AND PROTECTION TECHNIQUES

- ♦ Debridement
  - Nonselective debridement: Done with wet-to-moist dressings and wound/exposed bone irrigation using 19-gauge needle and 35-cc syringe
  - Selective debridement: Done with sharp instruments, focusing on removal of discolored, nonviable tissue
- ♦ Dressings
  - Wet-to-moist dressings with amphotericin B
- ♦ Topical agents
  - Topical application of amphotericin B

PHYSICAL AGENTS AND MECHANICAL MODALITIES

- ♦ The wound and exposed bone will be irrigated with amphotericin B using a 35-cc syringe and a 19-gauge needle. The medullary canal will be irrigated with amphotericin B using an infant feeding tube catheter and a 35-cc syringe. Physician orders were obtained for

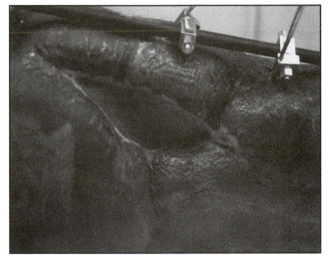

Figure 5-2. Right lateral thigh wound at time of home discharge. (See this figure in the Color Atlas following page 39.)

the use of this solution by the physical therapist due to this being a nonconventional form of treatment.

ANTICIPATED GOALS AND EXPECTED OUTCOMES

- ♦ Impact on pathology/pathophysiology
  - Bacterial/fungal burden is reduced (as evidenced by decreased fungal growth at time of next wound culture).
  - Debridement of nonviable tissue is achieved in 8 weeks.
  - Edema is reduced to WNL in 8 weeks.
  - Pain is decreased based on nonverbal signs to include decrease in facial grimaces and maintenance of HR during activities.
  - Physiological response to increased oxygen demand is improved.
  - Tissue perfusion and oxygenation is enhanced.
  - Wound size is reduced in 8 weeks.
- ♦ Impact on impairments
  - Integumentary integrity is improved as evidence by a decrease in nonviable/necrotic tissue and decrease in wound size.
  - Muscle performance improved.
  - Optimal joint alignment is achieved with appropriate positioning in 2 weeks.
  - Optimal loading on body parts is achieved.
  - ROM is improved, increasing within limits placed by orthopaedic surgeons.
  - Sensory awareness is increased.
- ♦ Impact on functional limitations

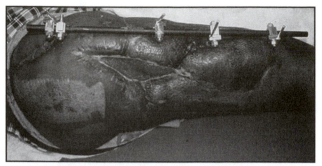

Figure 5-3. Right lateral thigh wound at time of 6-week follow-up appointment with MD. (See this figure in the Color Atlas following page 39.)

- Level of supervision required for tasks is decreased.
- Patient's ability to participate in activities related to self-care is increased.
- Performance of ADL is improved.
- Tolerance of positions and activities is increased especially tolerance of right hip internal rotation and right ankle dorsiflexion in positioning device in 3 weeks.
- ◆ Risk reduction/prevention
  - Protection of tissue is increased.
  - Risk of secondary impairment is reduced.
- ◆ Impact on health, wellness, and fitness
  - Disability is reduced.
  - Health status is improved.
  - Physical function is improved.
- ◆ Impact on societal resources
  - Accountability for services is increased.
  - Appropriate referrals are made to include nutrition, social work, and care coordination.
  - Decision making is enhanced regarding use of resources.
- ◆ Patient/client satisfaction
  - Care is coordinated with patient, family, and other professionals.
  - Coordination of care and communication are acceptable to patient and his family.
  - Patient and family knowledge of diagnosis, prognosis, interventions, goals, and expected outcomes is increased.
  - Patient and family understanding of goals and outcomes is increased.
  - Placement needs are determined and are acceptable to the patient and family.

REEXAMINATION

Reexamination is performed throughout the episode of care.

DISCHARGE

Mr. White is discharged from physical therapy after a total of 75 physical therapy sessions and attainment of his goals and expectations. These sessions have covered his entire episode of care. He is discharged because he has achieved his goals and expected outcomes.

> **Case Study #2:**
> **Sacral Pressure Ulcer**
> **Preop Free Flap Surgical Coverage**
>
> Mr. Charles Smith is a 74-year-old male who has a non-healing Stage IV sacral pressure ulcer (Figures 5-4 through 5-6).

PHYSICAL THERAPIST EXAMINATION

HISTORY

- ◆ General demographics: Charles Smith is a 74-year-old white male whose primary language is English. He is right-hand dominant.
- ◆ Social history: He is married and has three grown children and several grandchildren.
- ◆ Employment/work: Mr. Smith is a retired schoolteacher and football coach.
- ◆ Living environment: Mr. Smith and his wife live in a two-story home with four stairs to enter. There are railings installed on all stairs. Mr. Smith's bedroom is located on the second floor. Mr. Smith reports that he has a walker, wheelchair, and raised toilet seat at home.
- ◆ General health status
  - General health perception: Mr. Smith perceives himself to be in "poor" health since his bout with cancer 5 years ago.
  - Physical function: Limited to household ambulation and use of wheelchair for community negotiation.
  - Psychological function: He is depressed.
  - Role function: Husband, father, grandfather.
  - Social function: Mr. Smith and his wife both report that he enjoys social interaction with his family and friends. He enjoys watching his grandchildren play when they visit.

- Social/health habits: Mr. Smith does not smoke, drink alcohol, or use illicit drugs. He reports he is unable to exercise due to his physical condition.
- Family history: Both of Mr. Smith's parents had diabetes mellitus and HTN.
- Medical/surgical history: He has congestive heart failure (CHF), compensated cardiomyopathy (CMP), HTN, and atrial fibrillation. He had non-Hodgkin's lymphoma with radiotherapy and chemotherapy 5 years ago. Mr. Smith sustained a left hip fracture 2 years ago and underwent open reduction internal fixation (ORIF).
- Current condition(s)/chief complaint(s): Mr. Smith reports that he is in the hospital for treatment of a sacral pressure ulcer. The wound has been present approximately 18 months since the time of his inpatient rehabilitation post-hip fracture. He has pursued multiple treatment options including advanced wound care dressings, antibiotics, and hyperbaric oxygen therapy. However, he has not experienced successful wound healing. His plastic surgeon has recommended surgical closure of the wound. When asked if he has previously seen a physical therapist or nutritionist for this problem, Mr. Smith answered that he had not.
- Functional status and activity level: Mr. Smith reports that since his hip fracture 2 years ago, his mobility has been very limited by pain and "weakness." Prior to hospital admission, he was able to ambulate with a walker on level surfaces and used a cane on stairs. He required a wheelchair for long-distance locomotion. His wife assisted him daily with lower body bathing and dressing and with twice daily (BID) sacral wound dressing changes.
- Medications: On the date of physical therapy examination, Mr. Smith is on Unasyn, Prozac, Lasix, Coumadin, digoxin, Tylenol, and Percocet as needed (prn). Patient reports that these are the same medications that he was taking at home, with the exception of Unasyn (IV antibiotic) and Percocet.
- Other clinical tests
  - Lab values
    - Chemistry=WNL
    - Platelets=329,000/mm^3
    - WBC=6800/mm^3
    - Hct=29.6% indicating anemia
    - International normalized ratio (INR)=1.59
    - Partial thromboplastin time=34.7 seconds (normal=25 to 35 seconds)
    - Albumin=1.7 g/dL, no prealbumin data available
      - Normal albumin level is 3.5 to 5.0 g/dL, therefore a value of 1.7 indicates severe malnutrition
  - X-ray: Lumbar-sacral film negative for osteomyelitis

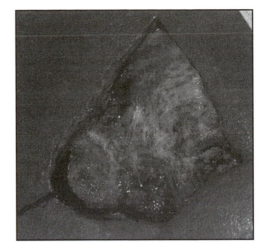

Figure 5-4. Sacral wound at time of initial physical therapy examination. (See this figure in the Color Atlas following page 39.)

SYSTEMS REVIEW

- Cardiovascular/pulmonary
  - BP: 130/74 mmHg
  - Edema: Absent, positive induration surrounding sacral wound noted
  - HR: 92 bpm
  - RR: 16 bpm
- Integumentary
  - Presence of scar formation
    - Healed surgical wound left lateral thigh at site of previous hip fracture ORIF
    - Decreased scar mobility noted in all directions
  - Skin color: Pale skin color throughout entire body
  - Skin integrity
    - Skin generally dry and thin-appearing
    - Open wound of sacral area surrounded by hyperpigmented skin and scar tissue, wound with significant drainage
- Musculoskeletal
  - Gross range of motion
    - LLE deficits at hip and knee
    - Decreased lumbar flexion in standing
  - Gross strength: Left hip musculature and quadriceps weak in comparison to other major muscle groups
  - Gross symmetry: Increased lumbar lordosis and mild left lateral lean noted in standing
  - Height: 5'11" (1.803 m)
  - Weight: 170 lbs (77.11 kg)
- Neuromuscular
  - Balance deficit in standing, requires bilateral UE support with assistive device to maintain static and dynamic balance

♦ Communication, affect, cognition, language, and learning style
  • Patient fully oriented and able to make all his needs known
  • Mr. Smith prefers to have instructions in writing and verbally to assist with his "memory"
  • Mild bilateral hearing loss noted
  • Mr. Smith does not own a hearing aid or eyeglasses
  • Mr. Smith's wife reports that after his hip fracture, depression limited his appetite and compliance with exercises
  • Mr. Smith reluctantly agrees and states that he is willing to be cooperative if it means that he will "heal"

TESTS AND MEASURES

♦ Circulation
  • Pulses: DP pulses palpable and equal bilaterally
  • Capillary refill
    ▪ 2 to 3 seconds in both feet
    ▪ Delayed at 3 to 4 seconds in hyperpigmented area surrounding sacral wound
♦ Cranial and peripheral nerve integrity
  • Tested using monofilaments as they are a reliable and valid tool for assessing light touch sensation[2]
  • Mr. Smith's vision is occluded and each of the following areas are tested three times
  • The monofilaments are applied with enough pressure to cause them to bend
    ▪ Plantar feet: He is able to perceive the 4.17 monofilament (1-gram pressure) on both feet
    ▪ Peri-sacral skin
      ▸ He is unable to perceive the 4.17 monofilament, therefore the test is repeated with the 5.07 monofilament (10 grams)
      ▸ He is unable to perceive this at least 50% of the time
      ▸ He is able to perceive the 6.10 monofilament 100% of the time
      ▸ Patient has loss of protective sensation in the peri-sacral area
♦ Gait, locomotion, and balance
  • Patient able to ambulate independently with walker x 100 feet on level surfaces
  • Antalgic gait and left lateral lean noted
  • Pain in area of left hip limiting longer distance ambulation
  • Patient requires minimal assist to maintain static standing balance without UE support
  • With UEs supported, he is able to stand without sway for at least 5 minutes

♦ Integumentary integrity
  • Peri-wound and associated skin
    ▪ Quality of skin surrounding the sacral wound is thin and fragile
    ▪ Assessment of hydration level reveals the skin is dry and scaly
    ▪ Hyperpigmentation is noted
    ▪ Area of discoloration extends 5 cm from wound edges, and color of the surrounding skin is reddish-brown indicating some degree of hemosiderin staining
    ▪ Raised and rigid scar tissue is observed at 50% of wound edges
    ▪ Firm pressure is applied to peri-wound skin to assess for edema
      ▸ The presence of induration, or firm edema, is noted
    ▪ Temperature of the peri-wound area is assessed in chronic wounds because an increase in temperature may reflect the presence of infection and a decrease in temperature may indicate a problem with vascular supply to the area
      ▸ Palpation may be qualitatively assessed via palpation with the dorsum of the therapist's hand and comparison to more proximal body segments[4]
      ▸ Palpation of the peri-sacral skin reveals no difference in temperature as compared to the lumbar or abdominal area
  • Wound (initial/preoperative exam)
    ▪ Location: Sacral
    ▪ Size: Direct measurement with a measuring stick=11.5 x 10 cm, central depth 2.5 cm down to sacrum
    ▪ Stage: Depth of wound is full-thickness according to the *Guide's* descriptions
      ▸ The universal pressure ulcer staging system (Table 5-4) is used here for improved communication with other disciplines and for compliance with the NPUAP guidelines
        ○ Mr. Smith's ulcer is a Stage IV[2]
  • Positions/postures that produce trauma to the skin/wound
    ▪ Pressure ulcers are most likely to occur over a bony prominence
    ▪ Mr. Smith is observed to be supine on the mat
    ▪ He states that he is uncomfortable in left sidelying due to hip pain, but that he does attempt to spend some time in right sidelying
  • Photography: Digital photographs are taken in order to document peri-wound and wound bed characteristics

- Anatomical structures: Sacral periosteum visible and fascia also noted
- Tunneling and undermining
  - A tunnel or tract is a narrow space originating in the wound bed that travels through the fascial layer
  - A probe was used to measure a 9.5-cm tract at the 4 o'clock position
  - Undermining is an erosion of the tissue at the wound edges
  - A probe was used to measure undermining: 2.0 cm at 12 o'clock, 1.0 cm at 8 o'clock, and 1.5 cm at 10 o'clock
- Tissue type: Wound bed characteristics are described
  - 30% viable fascia, sacral bone, and periosteum
  - 15% fibrous slough
  - 15% nonviable fat and hematoma
  - 40% pale, friable granulation tissue
- Drainage: Moderate serosanguinous
- Odor: Absent (assessed after wound irrigation)
- Signs of infection: Absent
◆ Muscle performance: Manual muscle tests
  - Hip flexors: R=4-/5 and L=3/5
  - Hip abductors: R=3+/5 and L=3-/5
  - Hip rotators: Patient does not tolerate resistance ≥ 3/5
  - Hip extensors: Weakness noted, patient does not tolerate test position
  - Quadriceps: R=4/5 and L=3+/5
◆ Pain
  - Patient rates his pain on the 0 to 10 NRS as 2 at rest and 5 with movement
  - The location of the pain is at the lateral left hip and mid-sacral area
  - He also reports that he is unable to sit longer than 20 minutes due to hip and sacral pain
◆ Range of motion: Measured with goniometer
  - Hip flexion: R=WNL and L=90 degrees
  - Hip internal rotation: R=WNL and L=10 degrees
  - Hip external rotation: R=WNL and L=15 degrees
  - Knee flexion: R=WNL and L=105 degrees
◆ Self-care and home management
  - Mr. Smith is able to ambulate to the bathroom independently using a walker and toilet himself using a raised commode with armrests (handrails)
  - Further self-care activities were not assessed
◆ Ventilation and respiration/gas exchange
  - SaO_2 96% on room air

EVALUATION

Mr. Smith is a 74-year-old male with a chronic, nonhealing, sacral pressure ulcer of 18 months' duration. His wound is full-thickness and is also classified as a Stage IV pressure ulcer because it extends to the bone. He exhibits impairments of the musculoskeletal system and the integumentary system. Functionally he is limited to short distance ambulation and has difficulty tolerating various positions due to pain, decreased ROM, muscle weakness, and integumentary disruption. The patient and his wife demonstrate a high level of motivation to meet the goals of wound healing and increased functional independence. His progress is expected to be limited by his nutritional status, the previous left hip fracture, and the effects of radiation.

Mr. Smith has a low serum albumin level, indicating protein deficiency. There is a correlation between low albumin and pressure ulcer severity.[3] It is anticipated that Mr. Smith will not have enough protein to heal after surgical intervention for his wound.

He never fully regained ROM, strength, and mobility after his hip fracture and is therefore unable to adequately change positions and provide pressure relief for the sacral area.

Five years ago Mr. Smith received radiation therapy for non-Hodgkin's lymphoma. Radiation therapy may cause injury to fibroblasts, injury to endothelial cells, and vascular damage. Skin that has been irradiated appears dry, hyperpigmented, thin, and fibrotic, much like the skin surrounding this patient's sacral wound. The damage done by radiation is

Table 5-4	
UNIVERSAL PRESSURE ULCER STAGING SYSTEM	
Stage	Description
I	Nonblanchable erythema, skin discoloration, edema, and induration
II	Superficial ulceration that presents as a shallow crater or blister; involves the epidermis and may involve a portion of the dermis
III	Deep ulcer that presents as a deep crater; involves epidermis, dermis, subcutaneous tissue; extends to but not through the underlying fascia
IV	Deep ulcer with extensive tissue destruction; involves epidermis, dermis, subcutaneous tissue, fascia, and underlying structures

permanent and may cause increased vulnerability to injury and delayed wound healing in the future. Irradiated skin requires protection from mechanical forces and from bacteria. His history of radiation was likely a factor in the development of his pressure ulcer and is expected to be a factor that may delay tissue healing.[3]

DIAGNOSIS

Mr. Smith has a chronic, full-thickness, nonhealing, sacral pressure ulcer with skin involvement extending into the bone and has pain in his left hip and mid-sacral area. He has impaired: circulation; cranial and peripheral nerve integrity; integumentary integrity; muscle performance; and range of motion. These findings are consistent with placement in Pattern E: Impaired Integumentary Integrity Associated With Skin Involvement Extending Into Fascia, Muscle, or Bone and Scar Formation. These impairments will be addressed in determining the prognosis and the plan of care.

PROGNOSIS AND PLAN OF CARE

Over the course of the visits, the following mutually established outcomes after surgery and at the end of this episode of care have been determined:

♦ Patient is able to more independently perform activities related to self-care and home management
♦ Physical function and quality of life are improved
♦ Wound and soft tissue healing is complete

To achieve these outcomes, the appropriate interventions for this patient are determined. These will include: coordination, communication, and documentation; patient/client-related instruction; therapeutic exercise; integumentary repair and protection techniques; electrotherapeutic modalities; and physical agents and mechanical modalities.

Based on the diagnosis and prognosis, Mr. Smith is expected to require between five to seven visits to prepare his wound for surgical intervention. Mr. Smith has malnutrition and a past medical history that includes irradiated skin and previous immobility due to a hip fracture. It is also recognized that the plan of care may need to be modified based on the success or failure of his surgical procedure.

INTERVENTIONS

RATIONALE FOR SELECTED INTERVENTIONS

Therapeutic Exercise

Mr. Smith will require a comprehensive therapeutic exercise program to address his impaired LE ROM and strength and his decreased balance. Flexibility exercises will assist Mr. Smith in regaining ROM in his bilateral hips and left knee. A strength training program of active exercise progressing to eventual resistive exercise will assist Mr. Smith in regaining gluteal and quadriceps muscle strength. Literature supports the use of strength training to improve dynamic muscle performance in elderly patients.[29]

Integumentary Repair and Protection Techniques

Debridement is indicated when there is foreign material or nonviable tissue in the wound bed. By selectively removing the fibrous slough from Mr. Smith's wound, his risk of infection will be decreased, and physical barriers to wound healing will be eliminated.[2] By choosing dressings that support moist wound healing, the proliferative phase of wound healing will be facilitated.[2]

Electrotherapeutic Modalities

Chronic wounds may benefit from electrotherapeutic modalities to facilitate the wound healing process. Mr. Smith has a nonhealing Stage IV pressure ulcer that has been unresponsive to conventional therapy. There is evidence to suggest that high volt pulsed current may improve the rate of healing in chronic pressure ulcers.[30]

Physical Agents and Mechanical Modalities

It has already been established that Mr. Smith has a chronic wound in need of cleansing and debridement. Pulsatile lavage with suction is a modality indicated for cleansing and debriding many wound types. It helps to remove necrotic tissue and exudates and to facilitate granulation tissue formation.[4] One study on patients with chronic wounds showed a higher rate of healing with pulsatile lavage as compared to whirlpool.[31]

COORDINATION, COMMUNICATION, AND DOCUMENTATION

The plan of care will be discussed and coordinated with the plastic surgery team. Once the patient's wound status is optimized with physical therapy interventions, he will be taken to the operating room for a latissimus dorsi muscle free flap to the sacral wound. This muscle should provide tissue bulk to fill the large defect. The physical therapist recommends that the nutrition service also be consulted preoperatively to address his malnutrition.

Wound care treatments will be coordinated with the nurse in order to ensure appropriate premedication and follow-through on wound cleansing and dressing procedures. Communication regarding the patient's functional and wound status will be communicated with him, his wife, and his nurse on a daily basis. All communication will be documented in the medical record.

The case manager will be contacted immediately regarding the probable need for short-term rehabilitation placement postoperatively.

PATIENT/CLIENT-RELATED INSTRUCTION

Mr. Smith and his wife will be educated regarding the plan of care and specifically instructed in:

- ◆ Infection control
  - The importance of decreased bacterial burden for successful wound healing will be explained
  - This is important preoperatively to prepare the wound for closure and also postoperatively to prevent postoperative flap infection[32]
- ◆ Flap precautions
  - In a free flap surgery, tissue is transplanted with its blood supply to the area requiring coverage
  - Using microsurgical technique, the blood supply of the transferred tissue can be connected to existing vessels at the recipient site so it can survive in its new location
  - Because of this delicate vascular repair, there are subsequent precautions that must be observed postoperatively to facilitate flap success[33-35]
  - The patient and his wife will be educated in these precautions:
    - Flap should be frequently observed for color
      - ▸ The color pink is ideal
      - ▸ Blue discoloration may indicate venous congestion and should be reported to the surgeon
    - Nurses, doctors, and therapists will check the flap for capillary refill
      - ▸ Ideally, capillaries will refill after 2 to 3 seconds of applying pressure
    - Nurses, doctors, and therapists will listen for Doppler ultrasound flow to more specifically check blood supply to the flap
    - Flap should be protected from any source of pressure or tension
    - The patient will be on a special low-air loss mattress and will need to avoid the supine position
    - He can expect to be on bedrest for 10 to 14 days in order to allow the flap adequate healing time
    - Even once healed, the flap will be at high risk for breakdown and must be vigilantly protected from shear, friction, tension, and pressure
    - The patient's wife will need to examine it daily for integrity and color change

THERAPEUTIC EXERCISE

- ◆ Balance, coordination, and agility training
  - Balance exercises will be performed during physi-

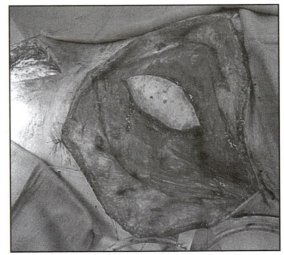

Figure 5-5. Harvest of latissimus dorsi free flap by plastic surgeon. (See this figure in the Color Atlas following page 39.)

cal therapy sessions to increase balance reactions in standing and decrease reliance on assistive device during gait
- ◆ Body mechanics and postural stabilization
  - Posture awareness training will focus on decreasing left lateral lean and increased tolerance of the standing position
- ◆ Flexibility exercises
  - Stretching exercises should be done after warming up, using a slow and steady stretch accompanied by deep breathing, and building hold up to 30 seconds
  - Mr. Smith and his wife will be trained in flexibility exercises with emphasis on increased left hip flexion and rotation and decreased hip/sacral pain
- ◆ Strength, power, and endurance training
  - The patient will be trained in isometric, active, and resistive exercises for the gluteals and quadriceps
  - A written program will be issued after training

INTEGUMENTARY REPAIR AND PROTECTION TECHNIQUES

- ◆ Debridement: Selective
  - Selective debridement with sharp instruments to remove nonviable tissue, specifically the fibrous slough
  - The rationale for removing this tissue is to reduce the bioburden of the wound, unmask any underlying exudate, restore circulation to the wound bed, and to allow for improved visualization of the wound bed[36]
  - If the wound does not respond to selective, sharp debridement, then debridement with an enzymatic agent may be considered

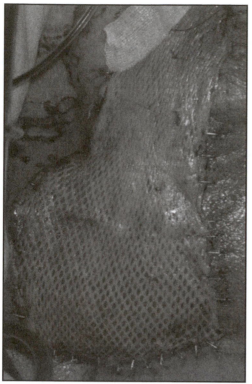

Figure 5-6. Sacral wound with free flap coverage. (See this figure in the Color Atlas following page 39.)

♦ Dressings
  • They should provide a moist wound environment to optimize healing potential
  • Fibroblast proliferation and collagen formation is known to be higher in a moist wound than in a dry wound[37]
  • An adherent semipermeable foam dressing will be used within the sacral wound to absorb moderate amount of drainage, provide cushioning over the bone, and at the same time maintain a moist environment
  • A skin barrier will be used to protect the periwound skin from moisture and adhesives
  • Dressings will be changed every other day during therapy sessions to allow for wound treatment and reassessment
  • Dressing may need to be changed by nursing sooner if it becomes saturated with exudate or rolls out of place
♦ Topical agents
  • Although the patient's wound is chronic and likely colonized with bacteria, it does not demonstrate any signs of wound infection at this time
  • Therefore, topical antimicrobial therapy will not be administered

  • If the wound does not demonstrate any response to the prescribed treatment within 2 weeks from the initiation of physical therapy, then a trial of topical antimicrobial therapy may be considered[32]
♦ Protective positioning program
  • A turning schedule with at least every-2-hour position changes will be posted in the patient's room
  • Pillows will be utilized as necessary to help maintain sidelying and decrease pressure on sacrum in supine
  • Head of bed (HOB) elevation above 30 degrees will be avoided

ELECTROTHERAPEUTIC MODALITIES

♦ Electrical stimulation
  • Is considered as a procedural intervention that may be appropriate in this patient's care
  • However its benefit may be limited due to short duration of treatment time prior to surgery
  • The use of electric stimulation peri-flap will need to be discussed with the surgeon postoperatively

PHYSICAL AGENTS AND MECHANICAL MODALITIES

♦ Pulsed lavage with suction is indicated in this case for thorough cleansing of the pressure ulcer and to facilitate irrigation of the tract and undermined areas[4]
  • This type of irrigation will facilitate nonselective debridement and subsequently help to loosen and remove fibrous slough from the base of the wound
  • Negative pressure from the suction may also help to improve the quality and perfusion of granulation tissue in preparation for surgery
  • The level of pounds per square inch (psi) may be modified based on his response and reported pain level during treatment
  • It should be noted that this intervention may be contraindicated postoperatively after the free flap to the sacrum

ANTICIPATED GOALS AND EXPECTED OUTCOMES

♦ Impact on pathology/pathophysiology
  • Debridement of nonviable tissue is achieved in 1 week.
  • Pain is decreased to 0 at rest and 2 with movement in 1 week.
  • Tissue perfusion and oxygenation are enhanced.
  • Wound inflammation is reduced and proliferation is facilitated as evidence by decreased signs and symptoms of inflammation in 1 week.

♦ Impact on impairments
  • LE muscle performance is improved by 1/2 muscle grade in all affected muscle groups in 2 weeks.
  • Postural control in standing is improved so that static standing is independent without sway for 5 minutes in 2 weeks.
  • ROM is increased by 10 degrees in all limited areas in 2 weeks.
♦ Impact on functional limitations
  • Tolerance of position changes is improved to 20 minutes for sidelying each side in 1 week.
♦ Risk reduction/prevention
  • Behaviors that foster postoperative wellness are acquired.
  • Pre- and postoperative complications are reduced.
  • Risk for further integumentary disruption is reduced.
  • Risk of secondary impairment is reduced.
  • Safety and physical function are improved.
♦ Impact on health, wellness, and fitness
  • Health status is improved.
  • Physical function is improved.
♦ Impact on societal resources
  • Appropriate referrals are made.
  • Documentation occurs throughout patient management and follows APTA's *Guidelines for Physical Therapy Documentation.*[1]
  • Intensity of care is decreased.
  • Placement needs are determined.
  • Utilization of physical therapy services is optimized.
♦ Patient/client satisfaction
  • Care is coordinated with patient/ family and other professionals.
  • Patient and family understanding of anticipated goals and expected outcomes is increased.
  • Patient's sense of well-being is improved by decreasing frequency of dressing change to every other day.

REEXAMINATION

Reexamination is performed throughout the episode of care.

DISCHARGE

Mr. Smith is discharged from physical therapy after a total of seven physical therapy sessions and attainment of his goals and expectations. These sessions have covered his entire episode of care. He is discharged because he has achieved his goals and expected outcomes. His wound is adequately prepared for plastic surgery closure.

Case Study #3: Electrical Wound With Free Flap Reconstruction

Mr. William Jackson is a 45-year-old electrician who sustained an electrical injury to his left wrist with resultant free flap reconstruction (Figures 5-7 through 5-9).

PHYSICAL THERAPIST EXAMINATION

HISTORY

♦ General demographics: Mr. Jackson is a 45-year-old white male whose primary language is English. He is left-hand dominant and is a graduate from a technical school.
♦ Social history: Mr. Jackson is married with two children at home.
♦ Employment/work: He works for the electric company as a high voltage technician.
♦ Living environment: He resides in a two-story home. There is one stair to enter without a railing and stairs to the second floor bedroom and bathroom with a railing.
♦ General health status
  • General health perception: Mr. Jackson reports that his health status is good.
  • Physical function: He was fully physically functioning in all activities prior to this accident.
  • Psychological function: Normal.
  • Role function: Husband, father, electrician.
  • Social function: He plays in a recreational softball league in the summer and a bowling league in the winter.
♦ Social/health habits: Mr. Jackson smokes one pack per day and classifies himself as a social drinker.
♦ Family history: HTN.
♦ Medical/surgical history: He had anterior cruciate (right) surgery 15 years ago. Otherwise his history is unremarkable.
♦ Current condition(s)/chief complaint(s): Mr. Jackson is 6 weeks post a latissimus dorsi free flap to his left wrist as a result of the electrical injury.
♦ Functional status and activity level: He is independent in transfers and ambulation. He has deficits with IADL using his LUE secondary to his recent surgery.
♦ Medications: Aspirin, multivitamin, Percocet.
♦ Other clinical tests
  • Lab values
    ▪ Hgb: 13 g/mL (normal 13.5 to 18 g/mL)
    ▪ Hct: 40% (normal 45% to 52%)

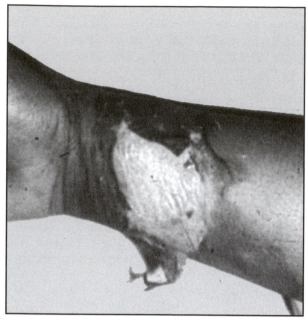

Figure 5-7. Right wrist high-volt electrical injury. (See this figure in the Color Atlas following page 39.)

■ Albumin: 3.0 g/dL (normal 3.5 to 5.0 g/dL)
■ INR: 1.8 (normal 0.9 to 1.1 when not on anticoagulant therapy)

SYSTEMS REVIEW

♦ Cardiovascular/pulmonary
  • BP: 124/68 mmHg
  • Edema: Moderate edema noted in the left wrist flap and digits of his left hand
  • HR: 76 bpm
  • RR: 12 rpm
♦ Integumentary
  • Presence of scar formation: Flap is in the maturation phase of wound healing
  • Skin color: WNL
  • Flap color: Pink
  • Skin integrity: Intact
♦ Musculoskeletal
  • Gross range of motion: WFL except left elbow, wrist, and hand
  • Gross strength: WFL except left elbow, wrist, and hand
  • Gross symmetry: LUE maintained in flexion
  • Height: 6'0" (1.83 m)
  • Weight: 180 lbs (81.6 kg)
♦ Neuromuscular
  • Balance: WFL
  • Locomotion, transfers, and transitions: WFL

♦ Communication, affect, cognition, language, and learning style
  • Communication, affect, cognition: WNL
  • Learning preferences: Visual learner

TESTS AND MEASURES

♦ Anthropometric characteristics
  • BMI: Weight (180 lbs) (81.6 kg) divided by height^2 (6') (1.83 m)=24.4 BMI placing Mr. Jackson in the normal category
♦ Circulation (see Table 3-4)
  • Pulse exam: 3+ radial pulses bilaterally
  • Palpable graft pulse
♦ Cranial and peripheral nerve integrity
  • Sensation: Mr Jackson had decreased two-point discrimination on his left hand and had significant loss of light touch and temperature over his flap
♦ Integumentary integrity
  • Inspection and palpation revealed no evidence of infection
  • Edema: 1+ pitting edema noted on the dorsum of the left hand
  • Circumferential measurements were taken of each digit at the DIP and PIP joints and at the proximal palmar crease and ulnar styloid process
    ■ Circumferential measurements provide the therapist with a quantifiable amount of edema and should be taken on both sides for comparison[2]
    ■ Results of circumference measurements in centimeters (cm)
      ▸ Thumb DIP=8, PIP (CMC)=11
      ▸ Index DIP=6.4, PIP=8
      ▸ Middle DIP=6.8, PIP=8.2
      ▸ Ring DIP=5.6, PIP=7.6
      ▸ Little DIP=4.8, PIP=5.6
      ▸ Distal palmar crease=25
      ▸ Wrist=31
  • Photography
    ■ Initial photos of the area were taken to assess healing over the course of therapy
  • Skin characteristics of flap donor site: Donor site was primarily closed and in the maturation phase of wound healing without evidence of infection or disruption
  • Scar: Vancouver Scar scale[38] (Table 5-5)
    ■ Mr. Jackson had a vascularity score of 2, a pliability score of 3, his pigmentation score was 2, and his height score was 2 for a total score of 9
♦ Muscle performance: WNL except for left elbow, wrist, and hand
  • Elbow 3/5 within available ROM

- Wrist 2-/5 within available ROM
- Digits 3-/5 within available ROM
- Orthotic, protective, and supportive devices
  - Mr. Jackson was in a protective wrist splint that was fashioned in a functional hand position
- Pain: 3 out of 10 on a VAS
- Range of motion: WNL except for his left elbow, wrist, and hand
  - Elbow flexion=20 to 100 degrees
  - Pronation=0 to 20 degrees
  - Supination=0 to 30 degrees
  - Wrist flexion=0 to 10 degrees
  - Wrist extension=0 degrees
  - Ulnar deviation=0 to 5 degrees
  - Radial deviation=0 to 5 degrees
  - MPs=20 to 50 degrees of flexion all digits
  - IPs=Limited to 10 to 20 degrees all digits
- Self-care and home management
  - He has some limitation with his self-care activities in the area of dressing and eating secondary to the injury being on his dominant UE
  - He was independent with bathing and toileting
- Sensory integrity
  - He had intact proprioception of his digits
- Work, community, and leisure integration or reintegration
  - Mr. Jackson has significant limitations in his performance of IADL secondary to his limited ROM and strength of his left wrist and hand
  - Mr. Jackson was not able to work due to his limitations at the time of his initial examination
  - Mr. Jackson was unable to participate in his leisure activities due to deficits in his dominant UE

EVALUATION

Mr. Jackson's history and risk factors previously outlined indicate that he is at risk for loss of left hand function as a result of an electrical injury with free flap repair. Mr. Jackson will benefit from a physical therapy program to decrease his impairments and increase his functional ability in an effort to return to his job as an electrician and his roles as a husband and father.

DIAGNOSIS

Mr. Jackson sustained an electrical injury with resultant need of a free flap repair of his left hand. He has pain in that hand. He has impaired: cranial and peripheral nerve integrity; integumentary integrity; muscle performance; and range of motion. He is functionally limited in self-care and

home management and in work, community, and leisure actions, tasks, and activities. These findings are consistent with placement in Pattern E: Impaired Integumentary Integrity Associated With Skin Involvement Extending Into Fascia, Muscle, or Bone and Scar Formation.[1] Placement of Mr. Jackson in this category is appropriate based on the extent of his electrical injury and the tissue repair performed which involves muscle. These impairments and functional limitations will be addressed in determining the prognosis and the plan of care.

PROGNOSIS AND PLAN OF CARE

Over the course of the visits, the following mutually established outcomes have been determined:
- Ability to assume or resume required roles is improved
- Ability to perform physical actions, tasks, or activities is improved
- Functional independence in ADL and IADL is increased
- Joint integrity and mobility are improved
- Muscle performance is improved
- Performance levels in self-care, home management, work, community, or leisure actions, tasks, or activities is improved

Table 5-5 VANCOUVER SCAR SCALE	
Vascularity Score 0 to 3	0: Normal 1: Pink (increase in blood supply) 2: Red (greater increase in blood supply) 3: Purple (significant vascularity)
Pliability Score 0 to 5	0: Normal 1: Supple 2: Yielding 3: Firm 4: Banding 5: Contracture
Pigmentation Score 0 to 3	0: Normal 1: Hypopigmentated 2: Mixed pigmentation 3: Hyperpigmentation
Height Score 0 to 3	0: Flat 1: <2 mm 2: 2 to 5 mm 3: >5 mm

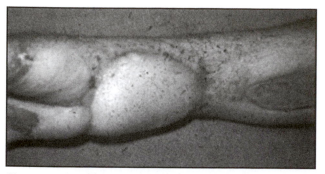

Figure 5-8. Right wrist electrical injury approximately 4 months post musculocutaneous free flap. (See this figure in the Color Atlas following page 39.)

♦ Referrals are made to other professionals or resources whenever necessary and appropriate

♦ Risk of secondary impairments is reduced (such as joint contractures)

♦ ROM is improved

♦ Sensory awareness is improved

♦ Soft tissue swelling is reduced

To achieve these outcomes, the appropriate interventions for this patient are determined. These will include: coordination, communication, and documentation; patient/client-related instruction; therapeutic exercise; functional training in self-care and home management; functional training in work, community, and leisure integration or reintegration; manual therapy techniques; prescription, application, and, as appropriate, fabrication of devices and equipment; and integumentary repair and protection techniques.

Based on the diagnosis and prognosis, Mr. Jackson is expected to require 75 visits over a 26-week period of time. Mr. Jackson lives with his wife and children, is motivated, and follows through with his home program. He is impaired, but is generally healthy.

INTERVENTIONS

RATIONALE FOR SELECTED INTERVENTIONS

Therapeutic Exercise

Exercise and functional activities are an essential component in the rehabilitation of the patient with a burn injury.[39] The goals of exercise for patients who have sustained burn injuries include a reduction in edema, prevention of contractures, preservation or increase in ROM and strength, and promotion of functional independence.[40] Exercise following burn injury and reconstruction may vary and may be physician dependent[41] requiring frequent communication to progress activities appropriately.

The various types of exercise may be broken down into three categories for the patient with burn injuries and include: ROM, conditioning, and functional exercises.[39] Mr. Jackson will require extensive work in the area of general ROM and functional exercises. PROM exercises are indicated to increase joint ROM and elongate soft tissue.[40,42]

AROM exercises are the preferred type of exercise to decrease edema, increase circulation, and to maintain and increase ROM and prevent muscle atrophy.[39,40,42]

Functional exercises should begin early in the course of burn rehabilitation and progress from basic ADL to increasingly more difficult activities.[39]

Manual Therapy Techniques

In conjunction with therapeutic exercise and the use of compression therapy, manual therapy techniques of soft tissue mobilization and massage are performed to facilitate edema reduction. Mobilization of scar can assist in the remolding phase of wound healing.[2]

Prescription, Application, and, as Appropriate, Fabrication of Devices and Equipment

Splinting is an essential component in the rehabilitation of the patient with a burn injury.[43] The use of splints offers protection, support, and positioning.[43]

Compression therapy is widely utilized in the treatment of burn scars[44] but the carryover to use with patients who have had flap procedures remains inconsistent. There continues to be limited studies as to the exact effect of pressure on scar formation, but it appears to decrease blood flow to the scar, which results in reduction of cell proliferation.[34] Pressure also appears to decrease edema in the area. In general it appears that compression therapy will enhance the maturation process[34] and should be considered in areas of deep dermal injury, skin grafting, and flap procedures.

Integumentary Repair and Protection Techniques

Moisturizers are frequently utilized in treating and preventing dry skin in patients with various conditions to include diabetes and burn scars.[2]

COORDINATION, COMMUNICATION, AND DOCUMENTATION

Communication will occur with Mr. Jackson's surgeon to address issues related to progression of activities based on flap healing. All elements of the patient's management will be documented.

PATIENT/CLIENT-RELATED INSTRUCTION

The patient will be provided information regarding healing and the impact of healing on deeper structures in relation to ROM, strength, and functional ability. Specific information regarding scar formation and contracture will be addressed to assist the patient in maintaining an active role in his rehabilitation program.

THERAPEUTIC EXERCISE

- ♦ Flexibility exercises
  - Stretching exercises should be done after warming up, using a slow and steady stretch accompanied by deep breathing, and building hold up to 30 seconds
  - ROM exercises of the LUE (elbow, wrist, and hand)
    - PROM
    - AAROM
    - AROM
    - Stretching exercises to increase tissue extensibility
- ♦ Strength, power, and endurance training
  - Progressive resistive exercise training with light weights and therabands

FUNCTIONAL TRAINING IN SELF-CARE AND HOME MANAGEMENT

- ♦ Self-care
  - ADL training to include dressing, grooming, and eating activities
  - Injury prevention or risk factor reduction with use of devices and equipment
    - Education in the signs and symptoms of pressure due to protective and supportive devices
    - Education in signs and symptoms of pressure related to compression therapies
- ♦ Home management
  - IADL training to include preparation for return to household chores

FUNCTIONAL TRAINING IN WORK, COMMUNITY, AND LEISURE INTEGRATION OR REINTEGRATION

- ♦ Work
  - IADL training to include preparation for return to work activities
    - Use of various tools required for his job as an electrician
    - Work simulation
- ♦ Leisure
  - IADL training to include preparation for return to leisure activities
    - Mr. Jackson progressively worked on grip activities required to hold a softball bat

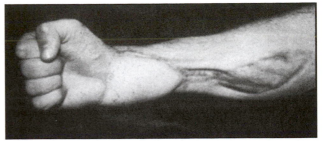

Figure 5-9. Right wrist electrical injury 1 year post injury. (See this figure in the Color Atlas following page 39.)

MANUAL THERAPY TECHNIQUES

- ♦ Mobilization of soft tissue
  - Retrograde massage to assist in the mobilization of fluid

PRESCRIPTION, APPLICATION, AND, AS APPROPRIATE, FABRICATION OF DEVICES AND EQUIPMENT

- ♦ Orthotic devices
  - Splint to maintain functional position and increase ROM
- ♦ Supportive devices
  - Progressive compression garments
    - Ace wrapping
    - Tubrigrip
    - Custom glove and sleeve

INTEGUMENTARY REPAIR AND PROTECTION TECHNIQUES

- ♦ Topical agents
  - Moisturizers
    - The use of moisturizers in full-thickness injuries and skin grafts is required secondary to the loss of naturally occurring skin lipids that were destroyed
    - The use of exogenous emollients is essential to decrease dry skin and prevent possible cracking and injury that can be a route of infection[45]

ANTICIPATED GOALS AND EXPECTED OUTCOMES

- ♦ Impact on pathology/pathophysiology
  - Soft tissue swelling, inflammation, and restriction are reduced to WNL in 6 months.
  - Tissue perfusion and oxygenation are enhanced.
- ♦ Impact on impairments

- Integumentary integrity is improved.
- Joint integrity and mobility are improved to manage complete hand grasp in 8 months.
- Muscle performance is returned to normal limits in 8 months.
- Optimal joint alignment is achieved in 1 month with appropriate night splinting.
- ROM is improved to WNL in 8 months.

♦ Impact on functional limitations
- Ability to assume or resume required self-care, home management, work, community, and leisure roles is improved.
- Ability to perform physical actions, tasks, or activities related to self-care, home management, work, community, and leisure is increased to independence in 2 months.
- Performance of and independence in ADL and IADL with or without devices and equipment are increased over the course of treatment with independence being achieved in 8 months.

♦ Risk reduction/prevention
- Risk of secondary impairments is reduced.

♦ Impact on health, wellness, and fitness
- Health status is improved.
- Physical function is improved.

♦ Impact on societal resources
- Referrals are made to other professionals or resources whenever necessary and appropriate, to include a referral to vocational rehabilitation.
- Resources are utilized in a cost-effective way.
- Utilization of physical therapy services is optimized.

♦ Patient/client satisfaction
- Documentation occurs throughout patient management and follows APTA's *Guidelines for Physical Therapy Documentation*.[1]
- Patient and family knowledge and awareness of the diagnosis, prognosis, interventions, and anticipated goals and outcomes are increased.
- Patient understanding of anticipated goals and expected outcomes is increased.
- Sense of well-being is improved as noted from increasing independence.

REEXAMINATION

Reexamination is performed throughout the episode of care.

DISCHARGE

Mr. Jackson is discharged from physical therapy after a total of 75 visits over 26 weeks and attainment of his goals and expectations. These sessions have covered his entire episode of care. He is discharged because he has achieved his goals and expected outcomes.

REFERENCES

1. American Physical Therapy Association. Guide to Physical Therapist Practice. 2nd ed. *Phys Ther.* 2001;81:9-744.
2. Myers B. *Wound Management: Principles and Practice.* Upper Saddle River, NJ: Prentice Hall: 2004.
3. McCulloch J, Kloth L, Feedar J. *Wound Healing: Alternatives in Management.* 2nd ed. Philadelphia, Pa: FA Davis Co; 1995.
4. Sussman C, Bates-Jensen B. *Wound Care: A Collaborative Practice Manual for Physical Therapists and Nurses.* Gaithersburg, Md: Aspen Publishers; 1998.
5. McCance KL, Huether SE. *Pathophysiology: The Biologic Basis for Disease in Adults & Children.* 4th ed. Philadelphia, Pa: Mosby; 2002.
6. Kucan JO, Brown R, Hickerson B, et al. *Plastic and Reconstructive Surgery: Essentials for Students.* Arlington, Ill: Plastic Surgery Educational Foundation; 1993.
7. Smith JW, Aston SJ, eds. *Grabb and Smith's Plastic Surgery.* 4th ed. Boston, Mass: Little, Brown and Co; 1991.
8. McGregor AD, McGregor. *Fundamental Techniques of Plastic Surgery and Their Surgical Applications.* 10th ed. New York, NY: Churchill Livingstone; 2000.
9. Biggs K, Driscoll J. Surgical interventions in wound management: practice considerations regarding skin grafts and flaps. Paper presented at American Physical Therapy Assocation Combined Sections Meeting: February 21, 2002; Boston, Mass.
10. Bergstrom N, Bennett MA, Carlson CE, et al. *Treatment of Pressure Ulcers: Clinical Practice Guideline No. 15.* Rockville, Md: US Department of Health and Human Services. Agency for Health Care Policy and Research; 1994.
11. Maklebust J, Magnan MA. Risk factors associated with having a pressure ulcer: secondary data analysis. *Advances in Skin and Wound Care.* 1994;7(6):25-42.
12. Maklebust J. Pressure ulcers: etiology and prevention. *Nurs Clin North Am.* 1987;22(2):359-377.
13. Berstrom N, Demuth PJ, Braden BJ. A clinical trial of the Braden Scale for predicting pressure sore risk. *Nurs Clin North Am.* 1987;22:417-428.
14. Johnson C. Pathologic manifestations of burn injuries. In: Richard RL, Staley MJ, eds. *Burn Care and Rehabilitation Principles and Practice.* Philadelphia, Pa: FA Davis Co; 1994:29-48.
15. Dimick AR. Emergency care. In: Hummel RP, ed. *Clinical Burn Therapy.* Boston, Mass: John Wright PSG; 1982:7-24.
16. Hummel RP. Triage and transfer procedures. In: Hummel RP, ed. *Clinical Burn Therapy.* Boston, Mass: John Wright PSG; 1982:25-34.
17. Lund CC, Browder NC. The estimation of areas of burns.

Surg Gynecol Obstet. 1944;79:352.

18. Wittman MI. Electrical and chemical burns. In: Richard RL, Staley MJ, eds. *Burn Care and Rehabilitation Principles and Practice.* Philadelphia, Pa: FA Davis Co; 1994:603-621.

19. Goodman CC, Fuller KS, Boissonnault WG. *Pathology Implications for the Physical Therapist.* 2nd ed. Philadelphia, Pa: WB Saunders; 2003.

20. Canale ST. *Campbell's Operative Orthopaedics.* 9th ed. Vol 1. New York, NY: Mosby; 1998:578-590.

21. Rockwood C, et al. *Rockwood and Green's Fractures in Adults.* 4th ed. Vol 1. New York, NY: Lippincott-Raven; 1996:147.

22. Johnson M, et al. Aspergillus: a rare primary organism in soft-tissue infections. *Am Surg.* 1998;64:122-126.

23. Denning D, Stevens D. Antifungal and surgical treatment of invasive aspergillosis: review of 2121 published cases. *Review of Infectious Disease.* 1990;12:1147-1189.

24. Gorbach S, Blacklow N, Bartlett J. *Infectious Diseases.* 2nd ed. Philadelphia, Pa: WB Saunders; 1998:936-938, 1339-1343, 2327-2332.

25. Gettleman L, Shetty A, Prober C. Posttraumatic invasive aspergillus fumigatus wound infection. *Pediatr Infect Dis J.* 1999;18(8):745-747.

26. Marcus J, et al. Extent of surgical intervention in primary soft-tissue aspergillosis. *Ann Plast Surg.* 1999;42:683-687.

27. Harden N, Luster S. Rehabilitation considerations in the care of the acute burn patient. *Critical Care Clinics North America.* 1991;3(2):245-253.

28. Jackson M, Flower C, Shneerson J. Treatment of symptomatic pulmonary aspergillomas with intracavitary instillation of amphotericin B through an indwelling catheter. *Thorax.* 1993;48:928-930.

29. Reeves N, Maganris C, Nanci M. Plasticity of dynamic muscle performance with strength training in elderly humans. *Muscle Nerve.* Jan 2005: e-published.

30. Griffin J, Tooms R, Medius R, et al. Efficacy of high volt pulsed current for healing pressure ulcers in patients with spinal cord injury. *Phys Ther.* 1991;71(6):433-444.

31. Haynes L, Brown M, Handley B. Comparison of Pulsavac and sterile whirlpool regarding the promotion of tissue granulation. *Phys Ther.* 1994;64(5):54.

32. Brown D, Smith D. Bacterial colonization/infection and the surgical management of pressure ulcers. *Ostomy/Wound Management.* 1999;45 (Suppl 1A):S109-S118.

33. Aston J, Beasley R, Thorne C. *Grabb and Smith's Plastic Surgery.* 5th ed. New York, NY: Lippincott-Raven Publishers; 1997:1030-1050.

34. Hallock G. Impact of the successful flap but failed reconstruction on the true rate of success in free tissue transfers. *J Reconstr Microsurg.* 2000;16(8):589-592.

35. Machens H, et al. Flap perfusion after free musculocutaneous tissue transfer: the impact of postoperative complications. *Plast Reconstr Surg.* 2000;105:2395-2399.

36. Gottrup F. Wound closure techniques. *Journal of Wound Care.* 1999;8(8):397-400.

37. Kerstein M. Moist wound healing: the clinical perspective. *Ostomy/Wound Management.* 1995;41(Suppl 7A):37S-43S.

38. Baryza MJ, Baryza GA. The Vancouver Scar Scale: an administration tool and its interrater reliability. *J Burn Care Rehabil.* 1994;15:181-188.

39. Humphrey C, Richard RL, Staley MJ. Soft tissue management and exercise. In: Richard RL, Staley MJ, eds. *Burn Care and Rehabilitation Principles and Practice.* Philadelphia, Pa: FA Davis Co; 1994:324-360.

40. Nothdurft D, Smith PS, LeMaster JE. Exercise and treatment modalities. In: Fisher SV, Helm PA, eds. *Comprehensive Rehabilitation of Burn.* Baltimore, Md: Williams & Wilkins; 1984:96-147.

41. Miller SF, Staley MJ, Richard RL. Surgical management of the burn patient. In: Richard RL, Staley MJ, eds. *Burn Care and Rehabilitation Principles and Practice.* Philadelphia, Pa: FA Davis Co; 1994:177-197.

42. Johnson CL. The role of physical therapy. In: Boswick JA, ed. *The Art and Science of Burn Care.* Rockville, Md: Aspen Publishers; 1987:299-306.

43. Humphrey C, Richard RL, Staley MJ. Soft tissue management and exercise. In: Richard RL, Staley MJ, eds. *Burn Care and Rehabilitation Principles and Practice.* Philadelphia, Pa: FA Davis Co; 1994:324-360.

44. Johnson CL. Physical therapists as scar modifiers. *Phys Ther.* 1984;64:1381-1387.

45. Poh-Fitzpatrick MB. Skin care of the healed burn patient. *Clin Plast Surg.* 1992;19(3):745-750.

Abbreviations

AAROM=active assistive range of motion
ABI=ankle-brachial index
ACE=angiotensin converting enzyme
ADL=activities of daily living
AHCPR=Agency of Healthcare Policy and Research (now
    known as the Agency for Healthcare Quality and
    Research)
AI=arterial insufficiency
AO/ASIF=Arbeitsgemeinschaft für osteosynthesefragen/
    Association for the Study of Internal Fixation
AROM=active range of motion
BID=twice daily
BLE=bilateral lower extremities
BMI=body mass index
BP=blood pressure
BUE=bilateral upper extremities
BUN=blood urea nitrogen
CEAP=clinical, etiologic, anatomic, and pathophysiolgic
CHF=congestive heart failure
CMC=carpometacarpal
CMP=cardiomyopathy
COPD=chronic obstructive pulmonary disease
CVA=cerebral vascular accident
CVD=chronic venous disease
DIP=distal interphalangeal
DMARDs=disease-modifying antirheumatic drugs
DP=dorsalis pedis
DVT=deep vein thrombosis
ECM=extracellular matrix
ESR=erythrocyte sedimentation rate
ET=endotracheal tube
FTSG=full-thickness skin graft
GARS-M=Modified Gait Abnormality Rating Scale
Hct=hematocrit
HCTZ=hydrochlorothiazide
HEP=home exercise program
Hgb=hemoglobin
HOB=head of bed
HR=heart rate
HTN= hypertension
IADL=instrumental activities of daily living
IDDM=insulin dependent diabetes mellitus
IM=intramedullary
IP=interphalangeal
IV=intravenous

LE=lower extremity
LLE=left lower extremity
LPN= licensed practical nurse
LUE=left upper extremity
MCP=metacarpophalangeal
MESS=Mangled Extremity Severity Score
MI=myocardial infarction
MRA=magnetic resonance angiography
MRI=magnetic resonance imaging
MS=multiple sclerosis
MTP=metatarsophalangeal
NPUAP=National Pressure Ulcer Advisory Panel
NSAIDs=nonsteroidal anti-inflammatory drugs
OA=osteoarthritis
OEE=Outcome Expectations for Exercise
ORIF=open reduction internal fixation
PAD=peripheral artery disease
PCA=patient-controlled anesthesia
PIP=proximal interphalangeal
prn=as needed
PROM=passive range of motion
psi=pounds per square inch
PT=posterior tibial
PVD=peripheral vascular disease
RA=rheumatoid arthritis
RLE=right lower extremity
ROM=range of motion
RR=respiratory rate
RUE=right upper extremity
SCI=spinal cord injury
SIMV=synchronous intermittent mandatory ventilation
SQ=subcutaneous
STSG=split-thickness skin graft
TBSA=total body surface area
TEE=transesophageal echocardiogram
TENS=transcutaneous electrical nerve stimulation
TIA=transient ischemic attack
TP=tibialis posterior
UE=upper extremity
UTI=urinary tract infection
VAS=visual analog scale
VI=venous insufficiency
WBC=white blood cell count
WFL=within functional limits
WNL=within normal limits

Brand Name Drugs and Products

The brand name drugs and products mentioned in this book are listed below, along with their manufacturer information.

DRUGS

Ativan (Wyeth-Ayerst, Madison, NJ)
Coumadin (BMS, New York, NY)
Demerol (Sanofi Winthrop, Gentilly, France)
Ditropan (Alza Corp, Mountain View, Calif)
Lasix (Aventis, Paris, France)
Neurontin (Pfizer Inc, Cambridge, Mass)
Nizoral (Janssen, Titusville, NJ)
Pepcid (Merck Sharp & Dohme, Whitehouse Station, NJ)
Percocet (Endo Pharmaceuticals, Chadds Ford, Pa)

Prozac (Eli Lilly & Co, Indianapolis, Ind)
Tylenol (McNeil Consumer, Fort Washington, Pa)
Unasyn (Pfizer, New York, NY)

PRODUCTS

Betadine (Purdue Pharma LP, Stamford, Conn)
Skin-Prep (Smith & Nephew, Hull, United Kingdom)
SensiCare (Inter-Decorativ-Cosmetic, Ohringen, Germany)
3M No Sting Skin Protectant (3M, St. Paul, Minn)

Index

WAIT

...There's More!

SLACK Incorporated's Health Care Books and Journals offers a wide selection of products in the field of Physical Therapy. We are dedicated to providing important works that educate, inform and improve the knowledge of our customers. Don't miss out on our other informative titles that will enhance your collection.

Essentials in Physical Therapy Series

The *Essentials in Physical Therapy* series answers the call to what today's physical therapy students and clinicians are looking for when integrating the *Guide to Physical Therapist Practice* into clinical care.

Essentials in Physical Therapy is led by Series Editor Dr. Marilyn Moffat, who brings together physical therapy's leading professionals to produce the most anticipated series of books in the physical therapy market to cover the four main systems:

- ♦ Musculoskeletal
- ♦ Cardiopulmonary
- ♦ Neuromuscular
- ♦ Integumentary

Written in a similar, user-friendly format, each book inside the *Essentials in Physical Therapy* series not only brings together the conceptual frameworks of the *Guide* language, but also parallels the patterns of the *Guide*.

In each case, where appropriate, a brief review of the pertinent anatomy, physiology, pathophysiology, imaging, and pharmacology is provided. Each pattern then details diversified case studies coinciding with the *Guide* format. The physical therapist examination, including history, systems review, and specific tests and measures for each case, as well as evaluation, diagnosis, prognosis, plan of care, and evidence-based interventions are also addressed.

Series Editor: Marilyn Moffat, PT, DPT, PhD, FAPTA, CSCS, *New York University, New York, NY*

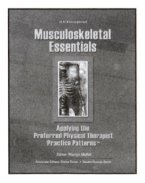

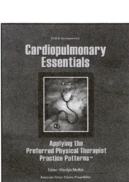

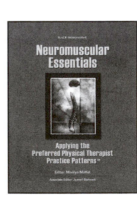

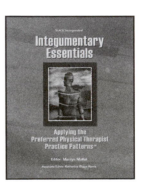

Essentials in Physical Therapy Series

Musculoskeletal Essentials: Applying the Preferred Physical Therapist Practice Patterns^{SM}
Marilyn Moffat, PT, DPT, PhD, FAPTA, CSCS, *New York University, New York, NY*; Elaine Rosen, PT, DHSc, OCS, FAAOMPT, *Hunter College, New York, NY*, and Sandra Rusnak-Smith, PT, DHSc, OCS, *Queens Physical Therapy Associates, Forest Hills, NY*
448 pp., Soft Cover, June 2006, ISBN 1-55642-667-4, Order #46674, **$58.95**

Cardiopulmonary Essentials: Applying the Preferred Physical Therapist Practice Patterns^{SM}
Marilyn Moffat, PT, DPT, PhD, FAPTA, CSCS, *New York University, New York, NY* and Donna Frownfelter, DPT, MA, CCS, FCCP, RRT, *Rosalind Franklin University of Medicine and Science, North Chicago, IL*
400 pp., Soft Cover, February 2007, ISBN 1-55642-668-2, Order #46682, **$58.95**

Neuromuscular Essentials: Applying the Preferred Physical Therapist Practice Patterns^{SM}
Marilyn Moffat, PT, DPT, PhD, FAPTA, CSCS, *New York University, New York, NY* and Joanell Bohmert, PT, MS, *University of Minnesota, Twin Cities, MN*
400 pp., Soft Cover, June 2007, ISBN 1-55642-669-0, Order #46690, **$58.95**

Integumentary Essentials: Applying the Preferred Physical Therapist Practice Patterns^{SM}
Marilyn Moffat, PT, DPT, PhD, FAPTA, CSCS, *New York University, New York, NY* and Katherine Biggs Harris, PT, MS, *Quinnipiac University, Hamden, CT*
160 pp., Soft Cover, June 2006, ISBN 1-55642-670-4, Order #46704, **$50.95**

Please visit

www.slackbooks.com

to order any of these titles!
24 Hours a Day...7 Days a Week!

Attention Industry Partners!
Whether you are interested in buying multiple copies of a book, chapter reprints, or looking for something new and different — we are able to accommodate your needs.

Multiple Copies
At attractive discounts starting for purchases as low as 25 copies for a single title, SLACK Incorporated will be able to meet all your of your needs.

Chapter Reprints
SLACK Incorporated is able to offer the chapters you want in a format that will lead to success. Bound with an attractive cover, use the chapters that are a fit specifically for your company. Available for quantities of 100 or more.

Customize
SLACK Incorporated is able to create a specialized custom version of any of our products specifically for your company.

Please contact the Marketing Manager of the Health Care Books and Journals for further details on multiple copy purchases, chapter reprints or custom printing at 1-800-257-8290 or 1-856-848-1000.

Please note all conditions are subject to change.

CODE: 328

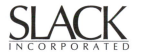

SLACK Incorporated • Health Care Books and Journals
6900 Grove Road • Thorofare, NJ 08086
1-800-257-8290 or 1-856-848-1000
Fax: 1-856-853-5991 • E-mail: orders@slackinc.com • Visit www.slackbooks.com